T0296421

FAST FACTS FOR THE CLASSROOM NURSING INSTRUCTOR

Patricia S. Yoder-Wise, EdD, RN-BC, NEA-BC, ANEF, FAAN, has taught in every type of nursing program from nursing assistant through doctoral programs and continuing education. Through The Wise Group, she and Dr. Kowalski provide consultation and development in teaching strategies, presentation and writing skills, coaching, storytelling, and leadership and management. Pat is a graduate of The Ohio State University, Wayne State University, and Texas Tech University. Currently, she teaches in the DNP program at the Texas Tech University Health Sciences Center and in the PhD program at Texas Woman's University–Houston. She is the writing coach for the University of Texas at Arlington and President of the Council on Graduate Education for Administration in Nursing. Her publications, including *Leading and Managing in Nursing,* focus mainly on leadership and management. She is the Editor-in-Chief of both *The Journal of Continuing Education in Nursing* and *Nursing Forum.* In addition to being a Virginia Henderson and Billye Brown Fellow (Sigma Theta Tau International), she serves as the cochair of the Strategic Advisory Committee for the state of Texas in its implementation of the Institute of Medicine report, *The Future of Nursing.*

Karren E. Kowalski, PhD, RN, NEA-BC, FAAN, has focused her career on the professional development of others, especially those on the front lines of care. Her work at Rush University, Centura Health Hospital, and Presbyterian-St. Luke's Hospital was geared to the primary role of leader in clinical areas. Throughout that time, and now through the Colorado Center for Nursing Excellence, she focused on preparing nurses for leadership and for teaching. Karren is a graduate of Indiana University, the University of Colorado Health Science Center, and the University of Colorado. She currently teaches in the DNP and master's programs at the Texas Tech University Health Sciences Center. Her publications focus mainly on leadership and management and include *Beyond Leading and Managing in Nursing,* which she coauthored with Dr. Yoder-Wise. She is an Associate Editor for *The Journal of Continuing Education in Nursing,* where she shares the Teaching Tips column with Dr. Diane Billings. Additionally, she serves on numerous editorial boards and review panels. She is the President and CEO of the Colorado Center for Nursing Excellence, where she serves as the co-lead of the Colorado Action Coalition, which is responsible for the implementation of the Institute of Medicine report, *The Future of Nursing.*

FAST FACTS FOR THE CLASSROOM NURSING INSTRUCTOR

Classroom Teaching in a Nutshell

Patricia S. Yoder-Wise, EdD, RN-BC,
NEA-BC, ANEF, FAAN

Karren E. Kowalski, PhD, RN, NEA-BC, FAAN

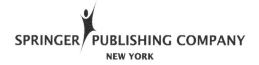
SPRINGER PUBLISHING COMPANY
NEW YORK

Springer Publishing Company, LLC
11 West 42nd Street
New York, NY 10036
www.springerpub.com

Acquisitions Editor: Margaret Zuccarini
Composition: S4Carlisle Publishing Services

ISBN: 978-0-8261-1016-9
E-book ISBN: 978-0-8261-0984-2

12 13 14/ 5 4 3 2 1

The author and the publisher of this Work have made every effort to use sources believed to be reliable to provide information that is accurate and compatible with the standards generally accepted at the time of publication. Because medical science is continually advancing, our knowledge base continues to expand. Therefore, as new information becomes available, changes in procedures become necessary. We recommend that the reader always consult current research, specific institutional policies, and current drug references before performing any clinical procedure or administering any drug. The author and publisher shall not be liable for any special, consequential, or exemplary damages resulting, in whole or in part, from the readers' use of, or reliance on, the information contained in this book. The publisher has no responsibility for the persistence or accuracy of URLs for external or third-party Internet Web sites referred to in this publication and does not guarantee that any content on such Web sites is, or will remain, accurate or appropriate.

Library of Congress Cataloging-in-Publication Data

Yoder-Wise, Patricia S., 1941–
   Fast facts for the classroom nursing instructor: classroom teaching in a nutshell/Patricia
S. Yoder-Wise, Karren Kowalski.
      p. ; cm.
   Includes bibliographical references and index.
   ISBN-13: 978-0-8261-1016-9
   ISBN-10: 0-8261-1016-9
   ISBN-13: 978-0-8261-0984-2 (e-book)
   I. Kowalski, Karren.   II. Title.
      [DNLM: 1.   Education, Nursing—methods. 2.   Faculty, Nursing. 3.   Nurse's Role.
      WY 18]
   LC classification not assigned
   610.7307'11—dc23
                                                                      2012004636

Special discounts on bulk quantities of our books are available to corporations, professional associations, pharmaceutical companies, health care organizations, and other qualifying groups.

If you are interested in a custom book, including chapters from more than one of our titles, we can provide that service as well.

For details, please contact:
Special Sales Department, Springer Publishing Company, LLC
11 West 42nd Street, 15th Floor, New York, NY 10036-8002
Phone: 877-687-7476 or 212-431-4370; Fax: 212-941-7842
Email: sales@springerpub.com

Printed in the United States of America by Hamilton Printing

Contents

Preface

Being an educator of nurses is a combination of two roles: nurse and educator. Either one by itself is challenging; together they can be daunting—or synergistic. The purpose of this text is to help both novice and seasoned educators gain skills in managing classroom experiences. Some of the ideas presented here can be applied in online courses; others are distinctive to the physical classroom where educators and learners interact. Most ideas can be used, with modifications, in large and small classes. They are ideas that work to keep learners focused on learning and not just occupying a geographic space.

The type of program itself doesn't matter in reading—and subsequently applying—the content of this text. The program can be a formal academic program resulting in a degree ranging from associate through doctoral. The content here also works in clinical conference discussions. It can work in formal programs such as ones of transition to the workplace (now more commonly thought of as residency programs) or ones of ongoing career development (commonly referred to as professional development or continuing education). These ideas work in any of those settings. The learners differ, the expectations differ, and the settings may differ; the techniques, however, are the same, even though they may be adjusted to more closely reflect the needs of a particular learner group.

For educators new to the field of teaching, this text can launch an opportunity for greater satisfaction and learner engagement. For educators established in the field, this text can provide some different strategies or ways of thinking about how the role of the educator facilitates or limits learners in their pursuit of new knowledge, skills, and attitudes. For administrative educators, this text provides new ways of thinking about educator competencies and what educators must do to help transform how learners learn.

Many educators learned to teach by watching someone else teach. The old "see one, do one, teach one" adage cannot meet the needs of today's learning environments and demands. Even without formal preparation as an educator, we must be able to employ sound strategies that keep learners engaged, move them toward success (however, that is defined within their educational pursuits), and help them use sound professional reasoning. The reason learners are engaged, move toward goals, and reason/think in a professional manner should be due to the educational interaction they experienced.

This text represents some of our best thinking about what educators can do to help learners learn and retain what they need to know to be effective. The text wasn't developed to be comprehensive. Rather, this text was developed to provide some key priorities on which educators need to focus in order to improve the learning experience. This text focuses on approaches designed to help learners grasp critical knowledge, skills, and attitudes; consider how learning develops clinical reasoning; and to value how learning will lead to better health care for the future.

Acknowledgments

We thank our husbands, who are always supportive of our endeavors and contribute to our richness of life. They make our work possible. They "fill in" when voids occur in simply managing life so that we can make this contribution to the profession. They see the humor in our silliness, they keep us laughing, and they are there for us during the tough times. We learn from them and then figure out how to translate that learning into meaningful experiences for those who are the recipients of our professional endeavors.

We would be remiss if we didn't acknowledge the "pioneers" in creating nursing education. Those range from Florence Nightingale to Adelaide Nutting to Rheba de Tornyay. Those are but a few of the names many of us can recall as making a distinctive impression on nursing education and how teaching is to occur. Further, some of today's great educators provided the quotes that begin each chapter. We are indebted to them for their thoughtful responses and timeliness. Thank you!

Over two careers, we have encountered many learners in many situations and have learned much from them. We too had role models of what a good educator could be and do, and we capitalized on all that we could learn from them. We learned what worked and what didn't from our colleagues and learners, and retested approaches. We know many other strategies exist, most of which we have used and many of which we still use. We figured out that good teaching is good teaching and it doesn't matter if the learner has zero prior knowledge about nursing or is a highly skilled clinical expert. Good teaching strategies engage learners, and that is the key to having a successful learning interaction.

Finally, we acknowledge that readers of this text have sought reinforcement for what they are doing or new ideas for what they could do. We appreciate your investment in making nursing education better. We invite your thoughts and feedback.

Patricia S. Yoder-Wise
Karren E. Kowalski

FAST FACTS FOR THE CLASSROOM NURSING INSTRUCTOR

The Nurse as Educator

I

Understanding Self

*A commitment to expanding knowledge of one's self
is a commitment to personal freedom, the choice to
take responsibility for the self one manifests to others.
Learners may forget the content and practice provided
by nurse educators; they will not forget the self the
educator made manifest.*

Phyllis B. Kritek, PhD, RN, FAAN

INTRODUCTION

*The most powerful tool educators have in the classroom
is what they bring of the self to the learning process.
Thus, educators need to understand themselves—
both their strengths and growth areas—through self-
assessment tools and reflection. In effect, educators are
leaders. When teaching in a classroom, for example,
the educators must lead learners to discovery so that
the knowledge is theirs. Understanding leadership
and themselves enables an educator to actualize effective teaching. To understand teaching tools and the use
of self enables educators to be effective in the classroom.*

In this chapter, you will learn:

1. The use of self as a valuable teaching tool
2. Available tools and insights to facilitate understanding self
3. The importance of leadership behaviors in the classroom
4. Development of characteristics of successful educators
5. The value of reflective practice

USE OF SELF

The primary tool the educator has when teaching in a classroom is *self*. Perhaps the easiest way to conceptualize the importance of self is within the *Emotional Intelligence* framework (Bradberry & Greaves, 2009).

In Exhibit 1.1, the quadrant focused on self-awareness is critical to the educator. Knowing and understanding one's self,

Exhibit 1.1   Emotional Intelligence

Four Quadrants of Emotional Intelligence

	SELF (Emotional Intelligence)	OTHERS (Social Intelligence)
AWARENESS	*Self-awareness*: knowing one's internal states, preferences, resources, and intuitions	*Social Awareness*: awareness of others' feelings, needs, and concerns
MANAGEMENT	*Self-management*: managing one's internal states, impulses, and resources	*Relationship management*: adeptness at inducing desirable responses in others

Source: Adapted from Goleman, Boyatzis, and McKee (2002) with permission from Pisanos (2011).

including the educator's strongest attributes, maximizes the learning that occurs in the classroom. In addition, knowing what areas of teaching are not so strong, and knowing how compensatory mechanisms or strategies are activated to adjust for these areas are vital to being successful. How well do educators understand their own internal states, what their preferences are, and the rationale underlying their preference? Self-awareness is a matter of asking what the internal motivations for specific behaviors are. Self-assessment tools that increase understanding, discussed later, are also available.

Self-Management

Self-awareness can lead to understanding how one handles or manages one's self in a variety of situations. Most of these situations, both the fun and the challenging, require both understanding and a willingness to practice whatever behaviors are needed to effect change. For example, being impulsive or cautious can serve different purposes and produce different outcomes. Asking what strategies might augment the positives and ameliorate or circumvent less desirable behaviors is valuable.

Social Awareness

How much are educators aware of the feelings, needs, and concerns of others? Becoming interested in others and curious about their specific behaviors and responses is the beginning of social awareness. This curiosity implies lack of negative judgment about the expressions and behavior of learners or even peers. Rather, a question is asked about what would make a learner do or say certain things or behave in specific ways. This action promotes understanding rather than criticism. Asking questions of the learner about specific behaviors creates understanding and can contribute to building meaningful relationships with learners.

Relationship Management

The relationship management aspects of emotional intelligence address the ability to work well with others and to utilize the understanding of self and others in subtle ways that induce desirable responses in others. For example, understanding upset as demonstrated by colleagues or learners in ways that do not make them "wrong" contributes to building successful relationships. In addition, this understanding allows educators to use tools to de-escalate difficult situations or upset responses.

═══════════════════════════════*FAST FACTS in a NUTSHELL*

- Use of self is the most powerful tool an educator has.
- Managing oneself provides the educator with more control.
- Being emotionally intelligent helps form positive relationships.

TOOLS TO FACILITATE SELF-UNDERSTANDING

Many tools exist to help individuals understand themselves better. The ones cited here are relatively inexpensive and readily accessible. They also have substantive data supporting their use.

EQ Map

The EQ Map (Essi Systems, n.d.) is an assessment of the major aspects of Emotional Intelligence. This tool can be completed in 15 minutes online (www.eqmaponline.com) at a nominal cost. The electronic report comes back via e-mail and informs the user at which level the responses were scored: optimal, proficient, vulnerable, or caution. Twenty categories are evaluated and grouped into five performance zones: Current Environment, Emotional Literacy, Competencies, Values and Attitudes, and Outcomes. For example, the two response categories in the Current Environment Zone are Life Pressures and Life Satisfactions. These response categories (Life Pressures and Life Satisfactions) estimate the amount of stress the educator is experiencing. Thus the amount of positive and sustaining activity is also estimated. Both aspects help to determine levels of stress in this zone. Included in the report, after each of the five zones, is a section detailing the specific activities that could help move any of the scores higher into the proficient or optimal zones. In other words, this tool supports the educator in developing self-awareness by making suggestions for ways to increase any of the low scores in the zones. More information is available on the website.

StrengthsFinder 2.0

StrengthsFinder 2.0 (Rath, 2007) discusses the importance of emphasizing people's strengths. This book, for a nominal cost, contains an envelope with an access code and a website address that allows the book owner to go online and complete the assessment tool. This tool can be completed in less than 15 minutes and the report is sent via e-mail. The most important aspect about the book is the case made to encourage us to spend time and energy on further development of areas of our lives in which we already excel rather than to expend extensive time and energy on our weaknesses. The research from the Gallup organization, on which the book is based, identifies that we will never excel at our weak areas; we will only be mediocre. Yet many cultures focus on correcting and emphasizing work on personal weaknesses. This tool also summarizes strengths and provides an activity exercise with suggestions for how the educator could expand upon strengths. The report identifies the top five strengths.

Example:

Educator A receives this report: "Input, Activator, Positivity, Learner, and Arranger." Each strength is discussed in depth and recommendations are made for how to enhance the strength.

Under "Input," the following observations were made: "People who are especially talented in the Input theme have a craving to know more. Often they like to collect and archive all kinds of information."

The individualized strengths insights include descriptions of how those strengths are exhibited. For example, for Input, Educator A received information including the following:

Instinctively, educators who have strong Input talent attempt to surround themselves with thinkers and place a special value on collegial conversations. Occasionally these conversations might supply the Input person with a new idea or a fresh perspective. Educators may not know at that moment how something that was discussed, read, or observed will lead to another discovery or insight but they like to ask questions and seek understanding. Perhaps the animated give-and-take that is enjoyed occurs when the "input person" is in the company of specific individuals. Because of these strengths these people may attempt to sharpen their methods for adding new words to everyday vocabulary as well as their academic or professional vocabulary.

Additionally, Educator A receives a list of ideas for action, including the following:

- Look for jobs in which you are charged with acquiring new information each day, such as teaching, research, or journalism.

- Partner with someone with dominant Focus or Discipline talents. This person will help you stay on track when your inquisitiveness leads you down intriguing but distracting avenues.

- Your mind is open and absorbent. You naturally soak up information in the same way that a sponge soaks up water.

- Identify your areas of specialization, and actively seek more information about them.

- Deliberately increase your vocabulary. Collect new words, and learn the meaning of each of them.

Because most educator evaluations follow a prescribed format, an educator might actively solicit additional feedback from learners on how to enhance strengths rather than "fix" weaknesses. Such a discussion could also lead to talking about what the learners' strengths and weaknesses are and where their focus ought to be. Learners could also employ these tools to assess their strengths and how they can be expanded.

═══════════════════════════*FAST FACTS in a NUTSHELL*

- Understanding self is the key to becoming an excellent educator.
- Understanding self allows the educator to focus on the learners.

LEADING IN THE CLASSROOM

Many leader behaviors can be observed in the classroom. Six of these behaviors are described here. The educator is the leader in front of the classroom with the learners. The educator is perceived as the expert, the one who either knows or knows how to discover. The educator leads the learner through the process of discovery. This work is accomplished by adhering to basic leadership principles. First, however, educators must work on leader behaviors and characteristics in themselves.

Create a Vision

Leaders create a vision through imagination and dreaming. They most certainly have dreams about how learners will be successful. Subsequently educators, the leaders in the classroom, identify strategies to engage learners in the vision of being successful. For most nurse learners, this is not a difficult task. It does require three specific educator strategies:

First strategy: Create a "brightness of the future" vision with the learner to assist the learner in "seeing" what they can have if they enroll in this vision.

Example:

Educator: How many of you would like to be a mediocre nurse?

Learners: [Probably no hands will go up.]

Educator: How many of you would like to be the best nurse you can be?

Learners: [Most likely all learners raise their hands.]

Educator: I am here to support you in accomplishing that goal. Everything that happens in this classroom is designed to help you reach that goal.

Second strategy: Employ a frequency of interaction. In addition to class time, create other opportunities to interact with the learner, such as office hours with the expectation that each learner set up at least one appointment with the educator. For staff development classes, one suggested opportunity is to foster conversations during breaks or after class. The focus is on creating relationships.

Third strategy: For learners to *truly* become enrolled, the third task is essential. It behooves the educator to identify any believable alternative to enrolling in the learning vision. In the example above, the believable alternative is to be a mediocre nurse—something almost no learner would want to be.

Build Trust

Effective educators build trust between themselves and the learners through the demonstration of specific behaviors. These behaviors include: accountability and responsibility, predictability, reliability, persistent behavior, and expertise.

1. The educator demonstrates *accountability and responsibility* with the learners.

    Accountability is the act of accepting ownership of the results or the lack thereof, while responsibility is defined as an obligation to accomplish a task or assignment. An activity that demonstrates this point might be a simple game of "Simon Says."

    ### Example:

    Educator: "Do you remember the rules for the game 'Simon Says'?"

    Learner: "You are to do what Simon Says. . . ."

    Educator: "Correct."

    "Simon Says, 'the game has begun.'"

    "Simon Says: 'Everyone stand up.'"

    "Simon Says: 'Clap your hands.'" (The educator claps hands overhead one time.)

    "and again." (The educator claps hands again.)

"Everyone who clapped their hands a second time, sit down. I did not say Simon Says." (This will probably be a major part of the class.)

"Simon Says: 'hop on one foot.'" (The educator hops once. Many will hop once and stop because that is what the educator did.)

"If you only hopped once, sit down." (Many more will sit down.)

"Simon Says: 'turn around.'" (Many will turn only once.)

"If you are not still turning, sit down." (A few learners will remain standing.)

"Simon Says: 'come to the front of the room.'" (Those people come forward and the educator can walk up and down the line. If at any time any learner smiles or says something, that person will have to sit down because Simon didn't say to do that.)

The educator does what he/she can to get as many to sit down as possible. And then acknowledges those who remain. Everyone claps . . .

The educator debriefs the game:

Educator: "How many of you in the first group to sit down thought to yourselves, 'The educator certainly wasn't very clear'?" (Some hands go up.)

"This is a demonstration of how we often think, which is 'laying blame' when the outcome isn't what we might want." (The educator leads a discussion of this behavior.)

"Did anyone think to themselves, 'I was up very late last night studying, I'm very tired,' and so forth? This constitutes justification." (The educator facilitates a discussion about justification.)

"Was there anyone who thought to themselves, 'Simon Says is a listening game. I was watching the educator rather than listening to what Simon Said'?" (The educator leads more discussion, which leads to accountable/responsible behavior.)

> "It is important to point out that most people spend time in all three places every day and we learn the most when we are accountable and responsible for both our thinking and our behavior, not from laying blame or justifying."

A game like Simon Says is a demonstration of principles that the educator would like to instill in the learner— accountable, responsible behavior. Leaders simply spend more time in the accountable–responsible level, learning from their experiences.

2. Another aspect of building trust is to be *predictable*. In the uncertainty of learning a new role, that of a nurse, the learners need stability. One way to achieve a strong, stable foundation is for the educator to be predictable. Teaching is not a guessing game. The learners should not have to guess "who" will show up in class today. Even educators who are predictably "bad" or really "tough" have demonstrated what is required for the learner to be successful. The greatest problem is for the educator to be unpredictable. This leads to uncertainty and causes distress that can manifest in challenging learner behavior in the classroom.

3. The educator must also be *reliable*. Reliability can translate into educators doing what they say they will do. If papers are promised to be returned on a certain day, the promise must be kept. When office hours are advertised to be a specific time, the educator must be in the office. Whatever rules or guidelines are promulgated, these rules must be honored by the educator as well as learners. Educators must role model doing what they say they will do. For staff development, the educator must do what is promised. This includes, for example, returning e-mails and phone calls or responding to requests in a timely fashion.

4. The educator needs to be *persistent*. This trait can be demonstrated as being unwilling to give up in difficult

situations. When obstacles appear, the educator role models, for the learners, strategies for overcoming the problems and issues. If there are difficulties with an examination, experiment, or class assignment, the educator can use questions to lead to a process of discovery or to determine alternatives. The educator does not give up.

5. Lastly, the educator demonstrates *expertise*. Even novice educators know considerably more than the learners about the content of the course being taught. This includes learners who have experience in other fields, such as Emergency Medical Technicians. It is not uncommon for these learners to believe that because they are competent at specific tasks such as starting IVs, the educator doesn't have anything to teach them. It can be valuable to demonstrate teaching expertise by asking questions about the foundation of the tasks, such as "What are the physiological underpinnings indicating the patient's need for an IV?" and then explaining why "The physician said to" is an incorrect answer. In these instances, understanding such situations demonstrates analysis rather than simple identification of the patient's situation.

Use of the above approaches to building trust with the learners demonstrates leadership in the classroom and the ability to create relationships.

Empower the Learner

Effective educators empower the learners to employ the necessary tools to become the best nurses they can be. They empower through encouraging the learners to stretch outside their comfort zones and practice new behaviors and thinking. They ask many questions to support learners in thinking through a situation or steps in a procedure. They encourage learners to take risks by doing things differently, but they are present to support the learners in this process. This is particularly valuable in simulation exercises where patient safety is not at risk. Be a cheerleader. Encourage learners in their efforts and find positives in the outcomes or the behaviors exhibited. Be positive and demonstrate that the educator believes that the learner can be successful.

Coaching

Effective leaders, and thus educators, focus on how they can coach learners through the learning process. Coaching means to direct, instruct, or prompt. It also means training intensely. In both the classroom and the clinical area, directing or prompting (often with questions that lead a learner through the process of discovery) is critical to the learning process. Because this skill is discussed elsewhere (Chapter 7, Coaching Learners), further depth is not provided here.

Getting Results

Educators focus on the outcome/result of supporting learners' processes. Often results are positive, especially when learners do well and respond to educators' efforts. Sometimes the results are not so positive when a learner is not doing well. Yet, educators convey that some of the best experiences came as a result of helping a learner see that nursing was not the best choice and that their particular skill set was better suited for a different career choice.

Sometimes results are measured in test scores. Great emotion can circle the issue of test scores and grades. When tests are viewed as a learning tool—an opportunity to correct misperceptions—the tests ought to be reviewed in class. Some structure around this process is helpful. For example,

the educator could provide specific directions for how learners challenge any of the test questions:

> *Educator:* If you have questions about the correct test response,
> email a reference/citation that disputes the designated correct
> answer. The reference must be more recent than the informa-
> tion used to substantiate the indicated "correct" answer. This
> reference/citation, from an approved source, must be received
> within 48 hours of the test discussion.

Educators may also choose not to review test questions. However, in reviewing the test statistics, the wise educator knows
what information to correct through discussion or some form
of feedback.

Guidelines such as these support a calm, reasoned discussion of differing opinions.

Acknowledgment

In most instances human beings, both educators and learners, are hardest on themselves. Both groups seem to have a
little voice in their heads delivering messages such as "You
certainly messed that up!" "You didn't do very well on that
response!" or "Notice the class laughed at you!" Focusing on
acknowledgments helps to shift that little voice. It is valuable
for educators to demonstrate being gentler with themselves
so that the learners have a role model for being gentler with
themselves. Educators can practice this skill set on themselves as well as using it with learners.

Likewise, educators who consistently use acknowledgment
of learners support them in gaining confidence and demonstrate the power of positivity. When the educator consistently
identifies what a learner does well, the learner's confidence
in the ability to perform skills and tools and to think critically about specific situations or issues grows steadily. Some
would say that people come to work to be acknowledged. Yet,

in nurse satisfaction surveys, acknowledgment by the supervisor consistently receives the lowest scores on the entire survey. Most educators believe they acknowledge learners "all the time." Somewhere a "disconnect" is evident. It may be how the acknowledgment is given. Guidelines for how to provide acknowledgment have been helpful for nursing leaders and may also be useful for educators. Exhibit 1.2 identifies some guidelines for consideration.

Exhibit 1.2   Guidelines for Acknowledgment

1. **Person to person.** Acknowledgments must be said to the person to whom you are grateful. Look the person directly in the eye. Take a moment, stop, look directly at them, and clearly state the acknowledgment. It also can be written. These can be kept, reviewed, and brought out whenever the person wants to remember the wonderful acknowledgment.
2. **Specific.** State exactly what the person has done that you appreciate. Do not just say, "Good job." Say specifically what he, she, or they did that was appreciated: "Thank you very much for completing the schedule for the next cycle. It looks fair, requests have been honored and all the shifts are covered."
3. **From the heart.** Acknowledgments must be "real." If it is a mere formality, do not waste your time because people know when the gratitude is not sincere. When this is the case, it is almost insulting. To continue, "Had you not helped

(continued)

Exhibit 1.2   *(continued)*

to finish the schedule, it would have been late coming out and staff would have been distraught. Your help was invaluable."

4. **Timing**. It is important to deliver the acknowledgment as close to the event as possible. The more time lapses between the event and the acknowledgment, the less sincere and heart-felt it seems.

5. **Public when possible**. Public acknowledgment has more power. It also lets everyone on the unit, for example, know what behaviors are valued by the leader.

Source: Reprinted from Yoder-Wise and Kowalski (2006), with permission.

Educators can use these guidelines with their colleagues as well, by creating a gentle little voice inside their heads that acknowledges them.

==============*FAST FACTS in a NUTSHELL*

- Be generous with acknowledgments.
- Use the six basic leader behaviors when demonstrating leadership in the classroom.

DEVELOPING THE CHARACTERISTICS OF EXCELLENT EDUCATORS

The characteristics of excellent educators constitute a role model for the profession. The really good news is that adults develop their characters and these characteristics each and every day. An educator/leader in front of a class demonstrates leader characteristics in several ways.

Character

The first of these characteristics is *character development.* Key work focused on what constitutes character was done by Guinness (1999). Character can be defined as what you think or what you do when no one else will know or find out. Factors that contribute to character begin with societal influences, including family, school systems, friends, and the work place, that have formed the educator's *values and beliefs.* Each human being is influenced by these factors. In addition, educators who are focused on character development have the *capacity for deep and lasting change.* When presented with the evidence that substantiates different thoughts, ideas, or behaviors, they are willing to shift their paradigm, to do things differently, or to incorporate a new "ah-ha" or realization that something has changed significantly.

Educators focused on character development demonstrate *moral accountability* to their stated standards, values, and beliefs. In other words, they are clear about when they violate their values. For example, if someone believes in honesty but does not hold learners accountable for violating the plagiarism contract established by the school, the educator is in violation of the espoused values. This doesn't build character; instead, it detracts from character development.

Those who are working on building character recognize their own *destructive behaviors* and just say "no." Many behaviors are simply "bad habits." For example, failure to meet deadlines for returning learner papers or in posting the grades does not model appropriate behavior and detracts from character development.

Those working on positive development are able to *forgive themselves and others.* Educators who hold grudges against colleagues are caught in a negative cycle rather than being able to forgive and let go of issues or problems. When a person feels hurt by something someone else has said or done, it is important to respond without resentment. When that same cruel, thoughtless person experiences something bad, the educator should not be gleeful or smug about the other person's misfortune. It is even more important to be able to *forgive self*. Although educators may think they need to be perfect, it is really important to let go of self-condemnation. Consistently, human beings are very hard on themselves, particularly if they tend toward perfectionism. Give it up, no one is perfect! Teaching is about the journey and doing the best one can. Even more, it is about *humility* and giving others credit. While educators facilitate learning, the process is *not* about the educator—it is about the learner. The learners deserve the credit.

Commitment

Commitment is about passion, a fire in the heart, a willingness to do whatever it takes to accomplish the goal. One cannot be totally committed sometimes. Passion, the foundation of commitment, is more valuable than talent or intelligence. When educators are truly passionate about nursing, the passion for patient care and for understanding healing and health care is conveyed spontaneously and consequently engages and excites the learners. To determine commitment and the corresponding passion, complete the following exercise:

> **Exercise:** The question is: If you won $25,000,000, tax free, what would you do with the rest of your life?

> **Debrief:** Keep in mind: You could build your dream house, provide college scholarships for family members and friends, give to charities, buy your dream car, take a trip around the world, and accomplish all of these adventures within 2 years. . . . So after this, what would you do for the rest of your life?

What have you always dreamed of doing? What would make your heart sing? What would challenge you to get up every day and work to accomplish a goal?

(For some people, this may not be nursing. That's OK. It is critical to NOT be on one's deathbed saying "if only I . . ." or "I wish I had. . . .")

Remember: Commitment is the will of the mind to finish what the heart has begun long after the emotion in which that promise was made has passed. Educators must ask themselves, "Am I committed to teach?" And learners must be asked, "Are you committed to nursing?".

Caring and Compassion

Leaders, and thus educators, simply care about more people. Educators have to care about their learners, each and every one. A part of this caring for the learners is remembering what it was like to be in their shoes. That might translate into making only reasonable assignments rather than assigning 6 chapters in the text and 10 additional articles per week. Caring can be interpreted as taking the risk of "being" with someone and sharing the complementary rhythm of suffering and joy. Learners have high moments experiencing the exultation of success and the low moments when the patient has a serious setback or even dies. They may question everything they did for the patient or hypothesize they could have done something better. The educator needs to ask appropriate questions and actively listen to the feelings of the learner.

Caring is giving of one's self and giving of one's time and focus. It is actively listening without other interruptions. It is being 100% focused on the learner and being completely present. Caring is about honoring the other person—seeing their wholeness, possibilities, hopes, and fears. Healing can emerge from caring.

Confidence

Belief in self and in what is being accomplished constitutes confidence. As a novice educator, confidence can be an issue. What stops confidence is FEAR.

Fear can cause the educator to "play it safe" so as not to lose or make an error rather than going for the "win," stretching outside the comfort zone, and attempting new behaviors. Additionally, fear distorts reality and makes things seem more dangerous; fear makes teaching seem harder or more difficult. Finally, fear can create a sense of desperation in which overcompensation looks like forced performance or delivery. Fear in the educator manifests in talking too fast, cramming too much information into a class, or filling the class with PowerPoint presentations rather than having discussions with the learners and discovering what they know. Confidence can translate into understanding clearly that even the novice educator knows more than what the learners know.

THE VALUE OF REFLECTIVE PRACTICE

Reflective practice is a powerful tool that supports the educator in continuing on a critical learning curve while teaching. It is a process of exposing contradictions in the practice of teaching. In exposing contradictions, the educator must first come to understand his or her own definition of the ideal educator. Then, the educator must examine the multiplicity of factors within the classroom interaction that either hindered or enhanced the educator's ability to achieve that ideal. While some educators can easily reflect on what happened in the classroom and on what they would do differently, one of the most useful methods of reflection for most educators is writing thoughts down, either in a journal or in a computer file. It can be quite valuable to be able to look back at the educator's daily or weekly observations when the course is completed. Those tools and strategies that worked, as well as those that didn't work so well, will be noted in the journal, which can lead to significant changes in educator behavior. The learning curve is enhanced by these discoveries.

═══FAST FACTS in a NUTSHELL

- Focus on understanding yourself.
- Identify those areas in which you can grow.
- Use tools such as reflection to track growth and change in teaching.

SYNTHESIS

Teaching effectively in the classroom demands that the educator have a clear understanding of self, a confidence that knowing oneself promotes creative and productive interactions with learners, and an ongoing reflection on how each class evolves using self-assessment that promotes a positive and effective learning process for the educator. Understanding self includes learning and growing every day, both in what the educator does in the classroom and in how the educator grows in character, commitment, caring, and confidence.

2

Role Modeling Being a Nurse

Learners gain a lot about the persona of nursing through observation of the professional behaviors exhibited by nurse educators teaching in the classroom. Professional behaviors such as caring, leadership, ethical decision making, critical thinking, and professional communications can all be role modeled during classroom interactions. Through positive role modeling, nurse educators have multiple opportunities to positively impact the professional development of future nurses.

Beverly Bowers, PhD, RN, CNS, ANEF

INTRODUCTION

Whether the educator elects to be an example/role model—or not—doesn't matter. The educator is the role model for the learners. The learners look to the educator for what a professional nurse is and what a professional nurse does. If the educator is passionate and excited about nursing and shows that to the learners, it makes all the difference in the world. If educators truly care about the learners and treat them with respect, they are modeling what exemplary nurses do, and the learners will carry that with them into their practice. No one gets up in the morning and decides to do the worse

> *possible job they can. Human beings begin with a strong desire to do their best, and it is the educator's responsibility to demonstrate what learners can discover about professionalism.*

In this chapter, you will learn:

1. How to role model professionalism
2. How to role model a passion for teaching, for the profession, for patient care, and for learners
3. The power of your attitude and positive reinforcement
4. The importance of preparation and practice
5. The importance of developing relationships with learners
6. How to role model being a functioning nurse

ASPECTS OF PROFESSIONAL ROLE MODELING

Learners are very aware of what the educator does. They are most apt to do what the educator does rather than what they are told to do. This natural human behavior only emphasizes the importance of role modeling that the educator demonstrates, often at an unconscious level.

Professionalism

A *professional* is a person who is paid to undertake a specialized set of tasks such as skill sets, good judgment, and polite behavior and to both implement and actualize them with caring and style. The most traditional examples of professions include medicine, law, and engineering. The term *professional* can also be used as a form of shorthand to describe a particular social stratum of well-educated workers who enjoy considerable work autonomy, a comfortable salary, and are commonly engaged in creative and intellectually challenging work. Because of the personal and confidential nature of many professional services and the necessity for their clients to trust them, most professionals are subject to strict codes of conduct that are derived from rigorous ethical and moral obligations. Nursing is viewed as a profession because it meets these expectations.

Attitude and Passion

The leadership research frequently addresses attitude for both the leader and the follower. Aptitude, including knowledge, skills, and intelligence, accounts for a relatively small amount of success; attitude, however, accounts for the vast majority of success. The wonderful news is that each of us chooses our attitude each and every day. Likewise, educators choose their attitude each day when walking into the classroom. Choosing a positive approach results in that approach being what the learners see. Being passionate is also visible to learners. Most of us began a nursing career with excitement, commitment, and a love for nursing and caring for human beings who are sick and in crisis. Learners today want that same passion for the profession, and they want to be challenged and acknowledged for work well done. They respond to educators who are passionate about their work and about patient care. In front of the classroom, educators have the opportunity to show learners passion and excitement about the specific topics and learning in general.

Sometimes educators, due to necessity, are assigned to courses for which they have little background or experience. In other words, they get the courses/classes that no one else wanted or they were least senior in getting their preferences. They might be given the notes from the educator who taught the course the previous semester. These notes could support receiving educator by identifying the details for the course and in looking for creative strategies for teaching the course. However, receiving educator might receive teaching materials that are densely focused on lectures and PowerPoint presentations. If such is the case, the receiving educator could use resources to incorporate different ideas by selecting a few of the lectures to refocus using a different approach. The rest of the lectures can be dealt with over time.

Exceptional educators radiate passion, conviction, and enthusiasm in their classes and their presentations. In a survey of business professionals, Koegel (2007) reported the number one characteristic of exceptional presenters is passion. This perception, no doubt, translates to most presentations and classes. If the educator is bored with the neurological system or doesn't understand it fully, neither will the learners. Thus learners will not be excited or engaged in the topic unless the educator is excited. If it is difficult to become passionate about a topic, search for a story or talk to colleagues about what they believe makes the subject exciting.

Appearance

How the educator looks is a reflection of professionalism. For example, the educator needs to be well dressed for the classroom, including well-maintained clothes, shoes, hair, and so forth. The educator must appear clean and neat with an air of confidence. In other words, look professional. The rule of thumb in presentations is for the presenter to dress one level above the audience. Because today's learners are quite casual, unless they are in some form of uniforms/scrubs, this rule may result in a look that is too casual for the purpose of role modeling professionalism. Most people have specific clothes in which they feel their best. Choosing those clothes on "teaching" days helps educators focus on facilitating learning rather than their personal appearance.

Appearance also includes such aspects as posture and body language. Stand up straight and command the room. Be confident. Even the inexperienced educator knows more than the learners about a specific topic.

Preparation and Practice

Be prepared for class. Nothing counts as much as preparation. Educators who are confident in their knowledge can focus on facilitation. Educators who are confident in both can focus on learners and their learning. Asking probing and stimulating questions can be difficult if the educator is not very familiar with the subject matter. Practicing how to share those aspects of the content that are provided in handouts or in a minimal number of PowerPoint slides is critical to feeling confident. Scenarios are an essential part of teaching, especially when the educator is striving to teach clinical judgment/critical thinking (Caputi, 2010). The days of 60 PowerPoint slides and a paper handout with each of the slides on the page are passé. According to Benner, Sutphen, Leonard, and Day (2010), using PowerPoint slides as a crib sheet or as a crutch for knowledge of the content does not support learning or the development of such skills as critical thinking and clinical judgment. Today's learners must have discussions of patient scenarios, experiential activities, and problem-solving exercises. Given the class time constraints, it is much better to limit the number of PowerPoint slides to a small number—such as a dozen—or to put the essential information in handouts. This design for class presentation requires both considerable preparation and practice presenting the content as well as extensive knowledge of the subject matter.

Professional Behavior

The educator must also demonstrate professional involvement. Because continuing learning and professional development exemplify commitment to the profession, these behaviors need to be role modeled for learners. For example, a discussion in class about membership in the National Student Nurses Association, assessing journal articles for their applicability, or practicing critical communication skills helps learners gain an appreciation for what professional nurses do.

Participation in professional organization activities models the importance of involvement in nursing organizations. Many of the clinically focused associations have either state or local chapters that provide continuing education related to the most recent developments, evidence, and research in the specialty. For example, the Oncology Nurses Association has very active state and local chapters that bring the latest research in oncology treatment and interventions to the practicing nurse (and they have a resource-rich website!). This is a group that has placed considerable emphasis on Oncology Certification that requires structured continuing education. Examining the standards of practice for specialty nursing groups also supports understanding the role of professional nurses and the responsibility they shoulder for implementing the best quality of patient care.

Journals and Journal Clubs

One of the easiest ways to stay current in a specialty role is to read the associated journals on a regular basis. This kind of information forms the basis for a monthly journal club that can review the latest trends in specialty practices. Providing the latest journal articles on a specific subject in the classroom conveys to the learners that continuing to read and learn are critical aspects of a professionally well-informed nurse. The learners are exposed to educators who look for evidence to update their practice and to ascertain the latest information about advances in patient care.

Writing, Publishing, and Speaking

Part of the expectations for professional educators is that they contribute to the literature through writing for professional publications such as the state nurses' association newsletter or for professional specialty or educational journals. If writing is not a personal strength, the educator can also speak publically on health care issues for community organizations, such as the Rotary or the PTA, or for the professional association. The educator can collect and share stories with the learners about these experiences. Such practices model the expectations of professional behavior for learners.

═══════════════════════════════════════ *FAST FACTS in a NUTSHELL*

- The passion and enthusiasm exhibited by the educator is critical to student learning.
- Looking and acting like a professional is critical for the educator to facilitate learners' development related to what it means to be a professional.

RELATIONSHIPS WITH LEARNERS

Liesveld and Miller (2005) identified that relationships are what drives the learning experience. They believe young people (and older people too) are thirsty for a caring adult or peer. Consequently, caring about learners and treating them with respect engages them in both learning and the profession. Some educators believe in doling out punishment, yet the experts believe that punishment kills learning and eventually corrodes the educator.

Demonstrating caring involves building a relationship with each learner. In extremely large classes this is difficult. Thus, educators need to develop strategies such as using assistants whom educators can nurture and coach. By role modeling what it means to be a nurse educator, educators might even influence those assistants to consider a career as a nurse educator.

Specific tools to develop relationships with learners include strategies such as memorizing learners' names. This can be accomplished by assigning seats or having the learners wear name tags with large letters. Making time for one-on-one meetings/discussions with learners also enhances relationships. Liesveld and Miller (2005) reported the need on the part of the learner for real human interaction in order to maximize learning. This report concurs with the position of Benner et al. (2010) in suggesting that the actual classroom experience is primarily interactive and problem solving rather than didactic lecture and PowerPoint slides.

Effective educators begin with conveying how important the learners are. This perspective is not an exaggeration because the learners are the future of the profession. They are the leaders and educators of tomorrow. Consequently their learning and their induction into the profession are highly influenced by the role models they see throughout the course of their learning.

Curiosity Versus Judgment

When a learner fails to study, does not do well on a test, or does not speak up in class, it is easy to make judgments about the behavior such as "the learner didn't study or take the time to work on the team project," "the learner is lazy and uninterested," or "the learner will never be able to function in the clinical area." Making judgments indicating that the learner is inadequate is easy and it is one approach to undesirable behavior. Another approach might be curiosity.

"What would make the learner not study?"

"What would prohibit the learner from active participation on the team?"

"What would make the learner appear disinterested?"

This thinking and the asking of questions about the learner are more productive and can lead to a creative strategy or intervention that may either help the learner alter behavior or may lead to redirecting the learner's interest. Either of these actions is preferable to judging the learner as "wrong," inadequate, or lazy.

Positive Reinforcement

The educator cannot provide enough positive reinforcement to learners. Learners are starved for the reassurance that they are progressing appropriately. The more verbal and nonverbal positive reinforcement that is provided, the better the performance from the learner and the better the relationship between the educator and the learner. Most educators can recall a specific educator who helped them develop as a nurse professional. No doubt, it was the educator who was the most positive about the progress being made. Attached to the positive reinforcement was the feeling that the educator really liked the learner. It is a natural connection that encourages the learner to work harder to create a cycle of receiving more positive reinforcement. Of course this serves as a key aspect in relationship development. If a respected figure clearly likes or "approves" of the learner, the behavior is likely to be reciprocated and will support the relationship and learning.

Educators can find at least one positive aspect for every learner and acknowledge the learner publicly. The classic research of Dr. Elizabeth Hurlock (1980), done in the early 1920's, was the first to document the power of public praise with grade school children. Learners seem to grow and bloom like flowers in time lapse photography with praise, both public and private, and with a relationship with the educator. That same response plays out across the life span. Providing positive feedback, demonstrating interest, and acknowledging the individual all contribute to developing learners.

Role Modeling Professional Thinking

Expert nurses give little consideration to how they walk into a patient's room and perform numerous related tasks. An expert may do all of the following quickly and easily: an overall patient assessment (including an emotional assessment), equipment assessments, an intravenous infusion assessment, an environmental assessment, and a safety assessment. Therefore, when teaching via the use of patient scenarios, the educator may ask questions that help the learner walk through a process such as one that a competent nurse would carry out. The educator is attempting to support the learner in the assessment process and to organize the acquisition of patient information in a reasonable and effective manner. Questions can lead the learner through the process of discovery and support them to think critically about the patient assessment process. Experienced educators may not be conscious of all the thinking that contributes to these assessments. Talking aloud about this process may assist in identifying the totality of the process. Sharing that process with the learners models the thinking behind the actions. In addition to gaining insight into the process of thinking critically and creatively, learners can value the actions that look relatively simple. Yet, they have important substance to make them appear so. Such an exercise models the process of professional thinking for the learner.

FAST FACTS in a NUTSHELL

- Relationships are the foundation for learning.
- Building a relationship requires praise, curiosity, and modeling.

SYNTHESIS

By role modeling the positive attributes of professional be-havior, a positive attitude, a passion for nursing and teach-ing, and by building relationships with learners, the educator can enhance the learners' experience and knowledge acquisi-tion. When role modeling, appropriate attire, mannerisms, and language, are necessary for the educator to demonstrate the ideal of not only how an educator behaves, but also how a nurse behaves. The educator can also demonstrate con-tinuous learning through professional involvement, reading, writing, and work in professional organizations. The educa-tor is consistently aware of the approach used with learners and focuses on curiosity and praise rather than judgment, as well as on building a relationship that honors each learner and supports them to be all they can be.

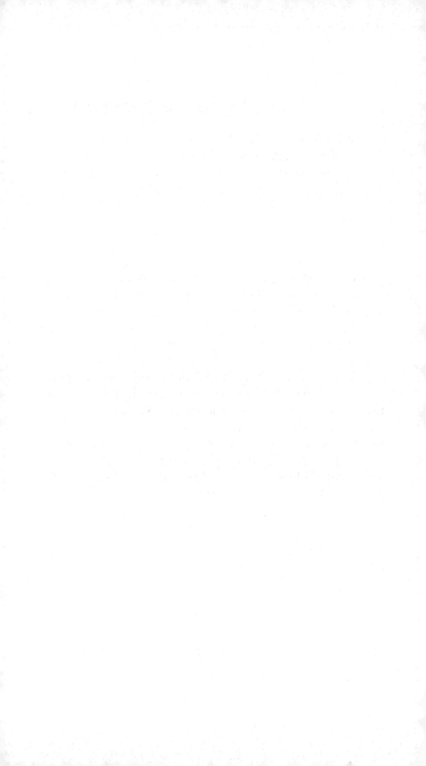

Setting the Environment
and Expectations

3

Preparing for the Classroom

Creating an effective classroom environment for learning is much like the process that nurses apply to create therapeutic environments in their other work settings. The nurse educator, in collaboration with learners, implements thoughtful and meaningful educational interventions based on a respectful assessment of learners and the purposes for their learning. In an energizing and encouraging atmosphere of shared expectations, every task seems easier and every learning goal seems more achievable.

Debra Hagler, PhD, RN, ACNS-BC, CNE, ANEF

INTRODUCTION

The crucial point about preparing to teach anything is to overprepare and prioritize. In other words, smart educators have additional resources available in case a discussion refocuses to some aspect of the topic that wasn't the most prevalent in the mind of the educator. An example of this might be having ready access to evidence about safety and quality issues related to the topic and the best evidence for nursing practice. Even thinking about what supplies educators commonly use in a classroom and putting them in a container to take to class can save time and embarrassment as well as serve as a safety net for the educator.

Simply recognizing it is not possible to cover all content about health care, the human condition, necessary nursing care, or the nuances of a disease condition can create a mindset that forces prioritization. Think about, for example, what is more common in acute care—cardiovascular procedures versus ophthalmologic procedures; or think about what is most critical or immediate, for example, critical interventions designed to save lives. These take priority in structuring class time. While the approach may seem harsh, acknowledging the importance of the topics not being discussed and alerting the learners to the reading materials where the content can be found serves as a reminder to learners. The key remains: overprepare, especially if the content has not been presented previously.

In this chapter, you will learn:

1. The importance of preparation for class
2. How organization is key to preparation
3. How practice instills confidence
4. The value of evidence and safety

CLASS PREPARATION

Preparation for teaching a course or a class begins with a self-assessment of the educator's current teaching skill set. Begin with the self-assessment tool in Exhibit 3.1. Reflecting on strengths is helpful and every educator has at least some. Reflect to an earlier presentation and what worked. One strength may be a warm, lovely, engaging smile. It is amazing how helpful this strength is for producing rapport and engagement with

Exhibit 3.1 Assess Your Presentation Skills

1. List three strengths about your presentations.
2. What are three skills you would like to begin working on this week?
3. Are you more comfortable presenting to learners or to educator colleagues?
4. What is the difference?
5. Are you more comfortable presenting when standing or sitting? What makes the difference?
6. Do you prefer a script, bullet points, or extemporaneous presentations?
7. Describe the responses of the learners to your class? Did they seem engaged?
8. Have you attended a course or a workshop focused on presentation skills?
9. Have you used video to assess your presentations? If yes, what did you learn?
10. Use this book, video, or a course and reevaluate your skills in 60 days.

the learners. As the assessment tool is completed, develop a plan for how to work on those skills that would benefit from improvement. Some helpful suggestions include:

1. Arrange to have your classroom presentation videotaped. Educators who have been videotaped and then critique themselves will have a clearer understanding of both the strengths and areas for improvement in their presentation.
2. Develop a plan for working on those aspects that require improvement.
3. Use the tools offered in this book.
4. Attend a course on presentations.
5. Continue to use videotaping to observe behavior.
6. Reevaluate progress in 60 days or after the last class.

Essential skills to use when teaching are listed in Exhibit 3.2. Both content and presentation style are identified in this list of approaches to remember. Each of the following requires pre-planning to create the environment that best facilitates learning. For example, in order to use learner names, educators must plan for seating charts or name tags to facilitate recall of learner names.

Exhibit 3.2   Skills That Promote Connecting to the Learners

1. Speak to what interests the learners.
   a. Learners focus on what they can use tomorrow. Create key points for content.
   b. Use the syllabus as a starting point.

2. Use your experience to create stories and examples; use anecdotes about coworkers.
   a. Begin collecting stories from clinical experience and from teaching other classes.
   b. See Chapter 9, Telling Stories.

3. Engagement requires eye contact. Look at the learners.
   a. Move around the room so that eye contact can be established with almost all of the learners.
   b. If possible leave the podium and walk down the aisles; move into proximity with the learners.

4. Smile.
   a. Even when the subject is serious, opportunities to smile exist. Smile when a correct response is given by one of the learners.

(continued)

Exhibit 3.2 *(continued)*

5. Use names often.
    a. Use name tags or tent cards to facilitate putting a first name with a face so learners can be called on by name.
    b. With a large group, a seating chart can be used to help with remembering names.

6. Use current references and journals.
    a. Using current references requires doing a quick literature search for the past 12 months to determine if any practices have changed.
    b. This demonstrates professional behavior.

7. Humor.
    a. Humor breaks down barriers and builds rapport.
    b. The educator is the primary source of humor.
    c. When educators make mistakes, using humor demonstrates humility and humanness.
    d. Tell funny stories (start your collection now).

8. Involve Learners.
    a. Ask questions.
    b. Use scenarios and have learners describe how they would deliver care and their rationale.
    c. Report the evidence as a part of the rationale.
    d. Identify possible safety issues and how these would be managed.

Using Course Syllabi and Class Objectives

The next key aspect of preparation begins with a review of the course syllabus or class objectives. Use these guidelines to decide which key aspects of the content to present and how to facilitate the discussion. If a file exists from the previous educator who taught the class, review the file. Begin with an outline of the key aspects of the class. For example, if it is a class on end-of-life care, the outline might include a background or history of the end-of-life care movement (hospice), the steps to be followed, the discussion with the patient and then with the family, the education of patient and family that is appropriate, and the process of facilitation of decision making in such situations. An outline is helpful to make certain that most aspects are covered. Then a story of an experience could be shared and scenarios created to serve as a foundation for the learner discussion.

Any didactic content should be limited and the majority of the time should be focused on the discussion by learners. Scenarios, which come from the personal experience of the educator or educator's colleagues, can be used to stimulate the discussion (Benner et al., 2010). Plan to involve the learners. The goal is to stimulate critical thinking and to develop clinical judgment. Use current references and evidence-based practice articles. Focus on the aspects of clinical practice that create a safe environment for patients and families. Don't forget to use humor and laugh.

Strategies to Engage Learners

Refrain from "calling" on learners. Doing this causes great anxiety and decreases participation. If some learners are not participating and discussion is primarily led by two or three learners, one strategy is for learners to take turns by going around the circle or down the row to answer questions. Using this approach avoids surprising learners, and they don't feel singled out and unable to respond.

===== *FAST FACTS in a NUTSHELL*

- Overprepare for the presentation.
- Analyze a self-assessment of teaching skills.
- Work to improve the teaching skills that cause discomfort.

PRACTICE, PRACTICE, PRACTICE

One of the most distracting and disengaging presentation styles is when an educator reads the prepared notes or Power-Point slides. What would make an educator choose this style? Perhaps that is the only way the educator has experienced presentations or teaching. Educators tend to teach the way they were taught unless they have additional information or experience. On the other hand, the educator may be unsure of the content and chooses this approach as a crutch to survive the class or presentation. It is no exaggeration to say that a class presentation must be practiced. Some educators prefer to nearly memorize the content. Others prefer to work from bullet points and some are more extemporaneous. Whichever style is selected, it is critical to know the material so well that the educator can actually "be" present with the learners. Being present with class learners translates into being able to:

- Watch for their reactions
- Notice facial expressions
- Notice who is engaged and who is not
- Note who participates and who does not

Knowing the content at this level allows for additional class-room creativity such as the use of games, dyads, or role playing.

Knowing the content enables the educator to be more confident. Practicing several times develops a honed style to allow the educator to open the space for creativity. Confidence, combined with enthusiasm about the class and a positive attitude, leads to a sense of "presence" that is telegraphed through the presentation. The implication is that the educator has a strong, positive demeanor or manner; the educator is poised with a strong bearing, carriage, and countenance. This approach translates into confidence by the learner that the educator is knowledgeable in what the educator says and shares. This result evolves from a willingness on the part of the educator to take the time to plan, organize, and practice. It conveys willingness by the educator to reflect and learn from each presentation or class that is taught. It can lead to a conversational style of presentation that enrolls the learners.

=========================*FAST FACTS in a NUTSHELL*

- Practice increases confidence and presence.
- Practice increases the likelihood of learner interaction.
- A minimum of three practice sessions improves the presentation.

EVIDENCE AND SAFTEY

Evidence-based practice and a focus on safe patient care are the current crux of educational efforts. It is vital to know, evaluate, understand, and implement the newest evidence that dictates nursing practice. This translates as a recent literature search for evidence of nursing care in the various disease entities being taught, such as congestive heart failure. The class needs to be constructed around not only the latest medical surgical textbook but also the recent research about the topic. A care plan can be constructed using this information. Some acute-care facility information systems have access to the last 12 months of literature on each diagnosis and a sample care plan. These could be included in class materials as examples for the learners.

The emphasis on quality and safety in patient care evolved from the Institute of Medicine report, *To Err Is Human: Building a Safer Health System* (Kohn, Corrigan, & Donaldson, 2000). Exhibit 3.3 provides the rationale for the intense focus on safety. For nursing, the *Quality and Safety Education for Nurses* (QSEN) project led by Cronenwelt et al. (2007) created a framework for the education of nurses at the undergraduate and graduate levels that focused on the knowledge, skills, and attitudes needed to provide safe care. For more information, consult the QSEN website (www .qsen.org). This framework for education is based on six elements:

- Patient-centered care
- Teamwork and collaboration
- Evidence-based practice
- Quality improvement
- Informatics
- Safety

The knowledge, skills, and attitudes needed by nurses are built into the educational curriculum. This is a demonstration of the importance of not only knowledge and skills but also the attitude or approach the nurse and the educator take to provide safe patient care. The essence of nursing is to keep patients safe.

Exhibit 3.3   Comments by Don Berwick in Conjunction With the Implementation of the 5 Million Lives Campaign

"The names of the patients whose lives we save can never be known. Our contribution will be what did not happen to them. And, though they are unknown, we will know that mothers and fathers are at graduations and weddings they would have missed, and that grandchildren will know grandparents they might never have known, and holidays will be taken, and work completed, and books read, and symphonies heard, and gardens tended that, without our work, would never have been."

Donald M. Berwick, MD, MPP
Former President and CEO
Institute for Healthcare Improvement

Source: Reprinted from Berwick (2006).

FAST FACTS in a NUTSHELL

- Educators teach learners how to keep patients safe.
- Commitment is demonstrated though the knowledge, skills, and attitude of the educator.

SYNTHESIS

If the standard for practicing nurses and nursing education curricula is focused on the knowledge, skills, and attitudes needed to provide safe care, how does this translate to the attitude or approach the educator needs to adopt when teaching a class or course? The attitude is demonstrated by the preparation, organization, and practice devoted to the knowledge and skills presented to the learners.

4

Creating and Using Agreements

*Agreements socialize the learners to the classroom.
They convey what our expectations are as an educator
and what our expectations of learners are. What is even
better is that well-developed agreements socialize
learners to professional behaviors they carry forward
in their careers.*

Suzanne M. Sutton, MSN, RN

INTRODUCTION

Educators frequently fear learners acting out in the
classroom. Many stories have been told where learners have demonstrated uncivil behavior toward peers
and educators in the classroom. Such difficult situations
can be averted with an effective yet little-used tool for a
smoothly running classroom. That tool is the class agreement. Most academic nursing programs have handbooks
that guide learners in comportment and acceptable behaviors and approaches. However, these guidelines are
rarely revisited or reviewed. To be effective, the educator must be clear with the learners from the first session
regarding expectations for both behaviors and outcomes.
Even if no one else uses agreements, any educator can
choose to do so.

In this chapter, you will learn:

1. The purpose of class agreements
2. How to construct class agreements to be discussed in the first class
3. How learners agree to the class agreements
4. How to hold learners accountable for these agreements

PURPOSE

The purpose of class agreements is to reach consensus with learners about how they will behave with each other and the educator while in the classroom. This exercise allows for a demonstration of what it means to make and keep an agreement. It also allows for the consequences if the agreement is not kept.

Because agreements provide structure, the class knows what to expect from the educator and from each other. Agreements are invaluable in managing the environment and demonstrating respect for each other.

=====*FAST FACTS in a NUTSHELL*

- Clearly identifying expectations supports learners to excel.
- Working to achieve a calm, smoothly running classroom supports all learners.

CONSTRUCTING CLASS AGREEMENTS

An example of a class agreement can be found in Exhibit 4.1. This is a beginning point and should be adapted to what the educator foresees as possible issues within a particular group. Content of the agreements can include expectations of

Exhibit 4.1 Example of a Class Agreement

ADMINISTRATIVE RULES

1. I understand that promptness is expected. I will be on time for the beginning of all classes and will return from breaks and meals promptly.
2. Further, I understand that I have committed to be present during the entire class.
3. I will turn cell phones to vibrate and will refrain from texting during class.

EXPLORATION, DISCOVERY, AND GROWTH RULES

4. I agree that all information shared by other participants will remain confidential. I will not repeat or discuss what is shared in class with anyone.
5. I agree that I will *not* engage in "sidebar" discussions.
6. I agree that I will direct my comments to whoever has the floor, whether it is the educator in the front of the room or a learner who is commenting.
7. I agree to participate verbally in discussions and exercises appropreately. It is my responsibility to weigh my fair share of contribution, speaking neither too often nor too little.
8. I agree to be open to new ideas and experiences.
9. I agree to take risks and step outside of my comfort zone.
10. I agree to maintain a positive attitude.
11. I agree to give supportive feedback and make corrections without invalidating anyone.
12. I agree to suspend judgment and be responsible for my actions.

(continued)

Exhibit 4.1   *(continued)*

13. I agree to be responsible for learning as much as I can from this experience. I also agree to ask for what I need from my educators and my fellow learners.
14. I agree to get better acquainted with my peers so we can all identify ways to support one another, work together as a team, and develop professionally.

ASSIGNMENT AND PROJECT EXPECTATIONS

15. I agree that I am responsible for completing assignments on time.

behavior in the class and expectations for timeliness in class and clinical arrival as well as in assignments and exams.

Begin with what would be valuable in class agreements. For example, consider what issues have disrupted learning in the past. Those disruptions often beg for an agreement to set a uniform expectation of what is acceptable. Once a set of expectations is developed, make sufficient copies so that each learner has a copy. The educator can retain a master copy that includes lines where all learners sign their names indicating they are in agreement with what is contained in the class agreements.

On the first day of class, the goal of the first housekeeping briefing is to review the draft of the agreements with the learners. This task includes a general statement or discussion of what makes agreements in the class important. The agreements convey a sense of openness and imply there are no hidden agendas or secret rules. This also allows the learners an opportunity to clarify or to amend the class agreements.

FAST FACTS in a NUTSHELL

- Consider past experiences of disruption as the basis for creating agreement statements.
- Assure that each learner has access to a copy of the agreements.
- Be sure each learner has the opportunity to sign the master document as a validation of being willing to be held accountable.

REACHING CONSENSUS ABOUT THE CLASS AGREEMENTS

To facilitate the discussion, the educator could have a different learner read one of the guidelines while the educator can provide clarity and ask if anything should be added or deleted. The educator could also ask learners, "Would you be willing to do the best you can with this agreement?" By allowing input and modifications, the educator conveys the sense of benefit to all and creates the potential for more learners to enroll in professional behaviors. If a statement is not negotiable, that point should be clear before providing opportunity for modifications.

The following information uses the examples of agreements found in Exhibit 4.1. After each agreement is presented, information related to the agreement is presented, including how to use it in the classroom.

Agreement Point 1:

I understand that promptness is expected. I will be on time for the beginning of all classes and will return from breaks and meals promptly.

Oftentimes a few learners do not understand the promise to arrive on time. They have multiple reasons such as baby sitters, weather, traffic jams, and so forth for why they cannot arrive on time. These may be the same human beings who will arrive late for the workplace. It is quite valuable to begin a professional career with a positive perspective and to begin this as learner. Arriving on time and starting class on time are important. Most likely everyone will indicate no problem about being on time. It is also possible to supply a cell phone number so that a message can be given to the educator and thus also to classmates when something untoward and out of the learner's control happens. Everyone then knows ahead of time an issue exists that the learner is attempting to problem solve. The educator can begin with having the learner apologize to the rest of the peer group and to the educator. If the late behavior persists, then other consequences can be assigned: a quarter in a piggy bank that the class can use for whatever they want at the end of the semester, points off a test, or the door can be locked and latecomers not admitted. This is a valuable discussion and emphasizes many aspects of professional behavior.

It is important to have both the guidelines and the consequences of failing to live up to the guidelines in the syllabus.

Agreement Point 2:

Further, I understand that I have committed to be present during the entire class.

Learners occasionally believe their needs supersede those of the educator or peers. They may believe it is acceptable to make personal appointments that require leaving class early without prior notification. Approval by the educator, on an exceptional basis, is the respectful approach.

Agreement Point 3:

I will turn cell phones to vibrate and will refrain from texting during class.

Cell phones ringing, especially with loud, fast-tempo music, can be quite disruptive to the class and educator. If they ring when a learner or educator is telling an important story, it can significantly disrupt the learning moment. In addition, the goal for class is to have learners prepared and interacting with their peers and the educator. Texting during class, playing games on a phone during class, or taking pictures are all unacceptable and essentially disrespectful of others. The learner has little chance to be engaged or to learn.

Agreement Point 4:

I agree that all information shared by other participants in class will remain confidential. I will not repeat or discuss what is shared in class with anyone.

Frequently, personal information is shared by learners in class. The goal is to make the classroom safe for learning. Thus, it is important that patient information and learner information not be shared outside the classroom unless permission is asked and received from the involved learner. These guidelines relate directly to *Health Insurance Portability and Accountability Act* (HIPAA) rules for patients and *Family Education Rights and Privacy Act* (FERPA) guidelines for learner privacy. On the other hand, the information shared by the educator is not part of this agreement, unless designated as such. Learners may share whatever the educators say with others outside the class unless the educator has specifically identified information as confidential.

Agreement Point 5:

I agree that I will *not* engage in "sidebar" discussions.

Sometimes classes are so fun or exciting that learners have difficulty containing themselves and speak out to their neighbors. This is understandable, yet leads to peers not being able to listen to whoever has "the floor." Without some structure and guidelines for the process within the classroom, chaos erupts. The educator may be able to handle sidebar conversations simply by walking over to the learners who are talking and standing by them. Most often they will stop talking. The educator could also ask those who are in the extraneous conversation if they have something they would like to share with the group. It is important not to ignore this behavior because soon the class will be out of control.

Agreement Point 6:

I agree that I will direct my comments to whoever has the floor, whether it is the educator in the front of the room or a learner who is commenting.

This agreement encourages orderliness in discussions and encourages people to be recognized when they have a comment or something to add. This agreement avoids everyone talking at the same time.

If several learners begin talking at one time, the educator may choose to stand very still in the front of the room and wait until learners become uncomfortable. Another strategy is to clap hands to gain the learners' attention. If it seems to be an ongoing problem due to the nature of the group, educators may choose to bring a bell, or a set of hand chimes or to use their phones to create a distracting noise.

Agreement Point 7:

I agree to participate verbally in discussions and exercises appropreately. It is my responsibility to weigh my fair share of contribution, speaking neither too often nor too little.

Every educator has had learners who monopolize the discussion time. They consistently have their hands up and other learners can become judgmental or impatient with these peers. Nearly every learner can identify another class or course in which they encountered a "monopolizer." It is very simple for the educator to ask a question such as, "How many of you have been in a class where one learner did almost all of the talking?" When the hands go up, the educator can explain to the learners that the goal is for all learners to participate. Educators can also use simple tools to assure balance in participation, such as going around the room in an orderly fashion and having the learners take turns in the discussion. Some educators draw learner names out of a hat or a basket. Many options exist to assure that all learners participate neither too much nor too little. Calling on learners randomly is not the best strategy as it puts learners "on the spot" and makes everyone anxious. This is not the best support for learning, nor is it respectful of the learner. Additionally, it decreases trust in the classroom.

Agreement Point 8:

I agree to be open to new ideas and experiences.

Although most learners act like sponges and are very open to learning as much as possible, some learners are challenged by their life experiences and have long-standing judgments about what ought to be done in specific situations. This can be a time when they are reminded about being open to new ideas. They can appreciate a different perspective.

Agreement Point 9:

I agree to take risks and step outside of my comfort zone.

It is easy to remain comfortable with what is "known," whether it is "the way we have always done it" or the way each of us was taught. Learning new ways to accomplish goals or achieve objectives requires the willingness to stretch beyond what we've known in the past and to try on new behaviors. It requires risk taking behaviors—the ability to attempt something new, something not done before. This new behavior can be both uncomfortable or anxiety producing AND very rewarding.

Agreement Point 10:

I agree to maintain a positive attitude.

Attitude is a powerful predictor of success. The good news is that human beings choose their attitude every day. For example, if three or more negative things happen in the morning getting ready for work, many people might see these activities as harbingers of what the entire day might become. The educator could relate a story about the morning:

> "The alarm didn't go off and I slept too late"; "I stepped on a child's hard plastic toy on the way to the bathroom and hurt a foot"; "I spilled the coffee and rushed around attempting to clean up"; and "I forgot some folders I needed for a meeting today and had to turn around and go back to retrieve them."

When three or more things go wrong as in this example, it might be easy to say "This is going to be a very bad day!" However, the reality is that human beings can choose to create the day differently even in the face of adversity. It is possible to smile and say, "I'm going to have a wonderful day!" The brain cannot take a joke and therefore believes the messages it receives. If negative messages are sent, the person has a bad day. If positive messages are sent, the day becomes more positive. Choosing a positive attitude is everything.

Agreement Point 11:

I agree to give supportive feedback and make corrections without invalidating anyone.

If the educator asks for a show of hands for the people who have received correction in a negative and demeaning manner, or "correction by crucifixion," the hand of almost every learner will go up. Everyone has received feedback in a destructive way. The goal for the class is that feedback be given in a constructive, supportive way. If this agreement is violated, the educator might ask of the learner, "Would you like to reframe the message?" and help the learner provide feedback that is thoughtful, kind, and supportive. Unhelpful feedback is usually about the negative tone and lack of respect conveyed rather than the actual words.

Agreement Point 12:

I agree to suspend judgment and be responsible for my actions.

Often judgment can be about a disagreement or difference in opinion or approach. It is most frequently tied to fear or pain/hurt. When learners are fearful or scared—which often derives from fear they won't be successful taking an exam, or even passing the *National Council Licensure Examination* (the RN licensing exam) (NCLEX®)—they make things and other people wrong, so they can be right. They have negative judgments about the educator, program, test, clinical rotation, or any situation that causes them to stretch or move into areas of the unknown.

Agreement Point 13:

I agree to be responsible for learning as much as I can from this experience. I also agree to ask for what I need from my educators and my fellow learners.

The unwritten implication is that the learners will study and come to class prepared for the discussion. They will do the best job they can in preparing for projects and tests. When they are unclear or uncertain, they will ask for assistance and support from classmates and the educators. They will utilize and implement what they learn in the classroom to function effectively in the clinical environment.

Agreement Point 14:

I agree to get better acquainted with my peers so we can all identify ways to support one another, work together as a team, and develop professionally.

Getting better acquainted supports the development of study groups and decreases the judgment of each other. It is easy to judge the person with whom you are unfamiliar. Some educators have learners identify one positive thing about each of their classmates.

Agreement Point 15:

I agree that I am responsible for completing assignments on time.

Educators can easily hold learners accountable for submitting assignments in a timely manner when this agreement is put in place at the beginning of the course. Doubtless, this agreement will avoid considerable hassle and negotiations for the educator.

It is very effective to end this part of the first session with questions such as: "Is there anything missing from these agreements that you would like to add?" "Is there an agreement you would like to change or you cannot live with during this course?" "Is everyone willing to abide by these agreements and do the best they can?"

Then, it is important to have each learner sign the document. This document is returned to the educator and kept for the duration of the course.

═══════════════════*FAST FACTS in a NUTSHELL*

- Agreements at the beginning of the course clarify expectations.
- They outline at the beginning of the course what is acceptable and unacceptable.

HOW TO HOLD LEARNERS ACCOUNTABLE FOR THE CLASS AGREEMENTS

The very first time a learner is late the educator must deal with the issue. The educator can suggest that an apology is owed to the class. If the tardiness continues, the educator can have a separate conversation with the learner to discover what the issues are for this person. The dialogue might proceed as follows:

> *Educator*: I noticed that you came to class late again today. What seems to be the problem or issue?
>
> *Learner*: I'm having problems with my babysitter. She arrives late and so I am late.
>
> *Educator*: We had an agreement at the beginning of class about timeliness. What is your plan to be able to keep your agreement?
>
> *Learner*: I really don't know what I am going to do. Do you have suggestions?
>
> *Educator*: Have you had a discussion with your sitter about the importance of arriving to class on time so that you don't miss important discussion or a quiz?
>
> *Learner*: I can do that.
>
> *Educator*: What would be your back-up plan if she continues to be late?
>
> *Learner*: I haven't thought that far ahead.
>
> *Educator*: Plan B is very helpful whether it is for a babysitter, for providing nursing care, or for taking charge of a unit. When would you be able to discuss a Plan B with me?
>
> *Learner*: After the weekend. Thank you for your help in thinking this through.

When the learner clearly works on the issue (tardiness) and arrives on time, privately acknowledge the improvement: "I noticed you have worked hard on a timely arrival for class. I appreciate your effort and the problem solving involved. Thank you."

Keeping track of the agreements for the first two or three class sessions sets the tone for the entire course. If the learners demonstrate behavior not consistent with their agreements, the behavior must be addressed if there is to be any hope of a smoothly functioning course. It is important that each learner remain calm, centered, and focused and not become frustrated or flustered. If necessary, practicing what to say to a learner with a colleague prior to discussion can increase the power of that communication.

FAST FACTS in a NUTSHELL

- Immediately address any violation of the agreements.
- Talk about the agreements in an open, calm, nonjudgmental manner.

SYNTHESIS

Making agreements and exhibiting a willingness to keep them is part of the maturation process. Holding learners accountable to the agreements they have made not only demonstrates the importance of accountability but also challenges all learners to the importance of abiding to the agreements, facilitating a smoothly functioning classroom.

5

Setting the Environment

Preparing for classroom activities takes a lot into consideration. In addition to the content and the specific learning activities, the wise educator takes into consideration the surroundings, both physical and social, and how they influence how the educator needs to prepare. Preparing has become increasingly complex in today's society as social and cultural forces that shape the life of a person or group have changed in an increasingly complex and global society. Today's classroom experience influences the engagement of learners and the outcomes of learning. That doesn't "just happen." The establishment of a comfortable learning atmosphere in early learner-educator interactions sets the stage for how learning is viewed.

Mary Lou Bond, PhD, RN, CNE, ANEF, FAAN

INTRODUCTION

Keeping the learners enrolled and engaged in the classroom is dependent on the environment created by the educator. Most educators can remember a course, class, or presentation that captivated them and held the participants spellbound. Since cell phones, texting, and computer games in class have already been addressed in the agreements, the focus of this chapter is on presentation skills that enroll and engage the learners. Educators are responsible for creating the classroom space, tone, culture, and expectations for the classroom. Likewise, they are responsible for observing the room and interacting with the learners in a way that creates a positive and exciting learning environment.

In this chapter, you will learn:

1. How to work with the space provided
2. Varying options for "setting" the room
3. How to create ritual
4. How to use silence

WORKING WITH THE SPACE

In large educational institutions, classrooms are frequently left in a state of disarray by the previous occupiers. The whiteboards or blackboards are not cleaned off and the chairs and tables are set in unsatisfactory ways. Trash may even be scattered around the room. While it is disconcerting to find a classroom in such a state of disorder, it is the responsibility of the educator to construct the classroom space in a way that reflects professional support for learning. If this means arriving early to clean and reorganize the room, then that is what is required. Remember two things: First, the room is a reflection of the educators. In other words, what the educator tolerates as acceptable is a reflection on them and their values. Second, the way the room looks is a reflection of the educator's respect or lack thereof for the learners. Respect for oneself and for the learners requires a clean, orderly room. This environment supports the learner in the learning process, because no distractions exist due to the room environment.

How to Set up the Room

Setting up the room depends in part on the size of the class. If there are 30 or fewer learners, the most effective format is setting the tables in a U-shape with the educator at the open part of the "U" (see Exhibit 5.1). This arrangement allows the learners to see each other and facilitates discussion. When there are greater than 30 learners, it may be necessary to seat the learners theater style. Due to room size and the number of learners, there may be fewer choices. However, that does not prohibit cleanliness and order. When a situation is difficult, some other strategies, such as bringing a potted flowering plant to relieve some of the austerity, may alleviate the institutional feel.

If the educator has considerable flexibility in how the room is arranged, that creates options. When using theater style, avoid arranging a rectangular room so that the educator is at one end and the learners stretch away from the speaker area. Remember that the educator can only interact with a limited number of learners when staying behind a podium (see Exhibit 5.2). It can be valuable to have notes and support material on a table and be able to walk down a center aisle and two side aisles to expand the number of learners that the educator can reach and with whom the educator can have direct eye contact.

Using the Space

In order to keep learners enrolled, it is necessary to be able to interact with them frequently. With small groups

Exhibit 5.1   U-shape Setup for 20–30 Participants

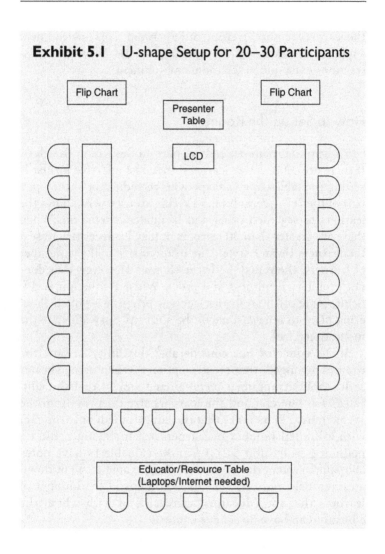

of learners, this is not difficult. Large groups of more than 30 learners (which is representative of most academic learning groups) will be more challenging. Approaches that could be used include:

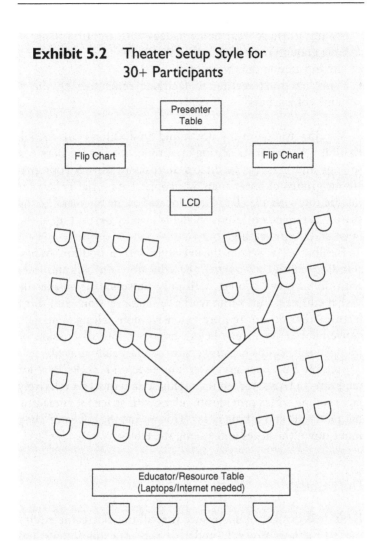

Exhibit 5.2   Theater Setup Style for 30+ Participants

- Moving around the classroom
- Speaking to one side of the room and then the other
- Breaking the large group into smaller groups for activities

- Having learners wear name badges with the first name large enough to be seen across the room
- Moving among the groups
- Using assigned seating to facilitate remembering the names of learners

Varying room setups are found in Exhibits 5.1 to 5.3. Exhibit 5.1 represents setting up a room so that learners can see one another; this facilitates discussion. This is appropriate for groups of fewer than 30 people. This setup is best for interaction with a leader who is located at the open end of the seating arrangement. Audiovisual is usually best set up at the open end of the seating.

Exhibit 5.2 is set up theater style with a podium. When standing behind a podium, the educator can communicate with or have eye contact with only those sitting inside the V-shaped lines. This setup works for large sessions and short lectures that do not require extensive note-taking. This is a convenient setup to use before breaking into discussion or role-playing groups because chairs can be easily moved.

Exhibit 5.3 is set up classroom style and works best for medium- to large-size lectures. This style requires a relatively large room. Tables provide attendees with space for spreading out materials and taking notes. This means the educator must move down the aisles and among the tables.

Electronics

Next, it is critical to make sure that all the electronic equipment functions properly and that the educator knows and understands how to use all the equipment. Having a specific contact in the technology or classroom support department is vital. Bring thoughtful treats or gifts to them. Frequently, the educator is fairly dependent upon this group and needs to build relationships with these technical support people.

Exhibit 5.3 Schoolroom or Classroom Setup for 30+ Participants

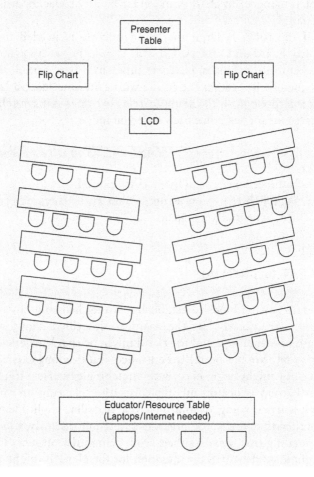

When Bill Gates introduced Windows 98, his computer shut down. This was a huge, important presentation. There was nothing but a blank screen and people scrambling attempting to get the electronics working again. If it can happen to

Bill Gates in a setting such as introducing "new electronics," it can happen to any educator. Always have a backup plan when using electronics. Identify what material can be presented using a flip chart or dry erase board or blackboard. Be prepared.

If the room is large and a microphone is needed to be clearly heard and understood, this should be set up prior to the beginning of class. Learners tune out if they cannot hear adequately. Be certain the sound works for you. Place a lavalier microphone so the sound carries but does not scratch or create extraneous noise each time you move.

═══════════════════════════════════*FAST FACTS in a NUTSHELL*

- Interaction between learners is optimal.
- Establish the room setup so that all learners can see, hear, and participate.

CREATING RITUAL

Creating ritual helps to establish a strong learning environment. Arrive early, set the room as described above, and **begin on time**. A part of the ritual might be that learners who arrive late are not permitted entrance. If it is a long class, the educator might begin class with stretching exercises. If it is a small group, educators might begin with a "clearing" in which each learner, going around the circle in order, might identify whether they are 100% present, and if not, identify what is happening that prevents them from being fully present. They might also identify their intention for the class. It might also be possible to ask if they have completed the required reading so that they can all have discussions rather than a lecture from a PowerPoint presentation.

In order to encourage critical thinking, the educator might have assigned a study sheet/handout and the ritual might be that the completed sheet would be the pass for admission to class (Benner et al., 2010). This facilitates the educator's ability to discuss the assignment with the learners rather than having to spoon feed the content to them.

One ritual might occur at the beginning of the course. The educator could systematically explain the syllabus, including the high standards and expectations of the learners. The educator could then reassure them by demonstrating confidence that all the learners can meet the standards. Such expectations support learners to excel and to do their very best.

Ritual could also be established around how tests are debriefed and what behavior is acceptable. "Rules" or expectations could also be assigned concerning how test questions can be challenged.

====*FAST FACTS in a NUTSHELL*

- Ritual has value for creating the environmental context.

RESPONSIBILITY/ACCOUNTABILITY

Nurses are responsible for patient safety and for the quality of care they deliver. This is a critical lesson for learners. Learners are responsible for completing all assignments and papers and for turning them in on time. They are responsible for completing these assignments in a manner that adheres to all the rules and guidelines concerning appropriate citations, use of the Internet, and plagiarism. If learners choose not to be responsible, they should be accountable for the consequences. Often consequences are identified in handbooks provided by the school. If the accountability is related to the class agreements (see Chapter 4), the consequences may be agreed upon by the group of learners and the educator together.

==*FAST FACTS in a NUTSHELL*

- Responsibility is key to the safe care of patients.

USE OF SILENCE

In the US culture, silence creates great discomfort. Few people can withstand silence. The automatic response is to fill the silence by speaking. This cultural trait can be used to the advantage of learners and educators. For example, when asking a question, it is important that the educator NOT jump into the silence with a follow-up question or, even more counterproductive, the answer. Rather, the educator asks a question and then waits, silently counting by thousands from 1 to 10: "One thousand and one, one thousand and two, . . ." until "one thousand and ten." The educator will usually not reach 10 before a learner will speak up. This is a strategy that supports learner participation and discussion, which is the goal of the classroom environment. If no response is provided, the educator can ask a more basic question to help learners build up to the initial question.

SYNTHESIS

Creating an environment in the classroom that honors and respects the learners as well as the educator sets the stage for an appropriate structure that facilitates and supports learning. Ritual provides comfort and familiarity for what is expected. Such efforts serve both learners and educators. Learners feel valued and the environment supports the educational process and allows the educator to do the best teaching possible.

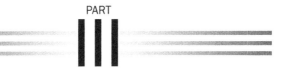

PART

III

Core Classroom Strategies

6

Engaging Learners

*Engaging today's nursing learner in class is quite
challenging, because many younger learners have
become used to fast-paced, varied activities that
"entertain." The "talking head" is soon tuned out.
My favorite lecture involves setting up a large display
of disaster preparedness supplies (e.g., flashlights,
emergency radios, non-perishable food, etc.) in front
of the room. As learners enter, I invite them to view
the items on the tables, then begin to discuss how
to make a plan and build a disaster supply kit. The
display items maintain their attention and stimulate
their imaginations about what they would put into
their own kit. Granted, not every lecture lends itself to
such a display, but we should try to identify strategies
to capture the attention of learners whenever possible.
The more senses we stimulate during class, the longer
new knowledge will be retained.*

Cheryl K. Schmidt, PhD, RN, CNE, ANEF

INTRODUCTION

Since Benner et al. (2010) have strongly encouraged educators to give up PowerPoints and use other strategies to teach learners, the question becomes, what other strategies do we use? This chapter is filled with tools regarding how to teach learners and keep them engaged in the topic. If names and structure are assigned to the behavioral aspects of teaching, it simplifies the ability to evaluate what worked in the teaching modality and didn't work. Understanding and utilizing these named strategies requires creativity and innovation. However, educators can build upon some of the examples provided in this chapter to expand their ability to engage learners.

In this chapter, you will learn:

1. Tools that engage the learner
2. How to open a course or class in an engaging manner that captures attention
3. Key concepts that create the classroom environment, including participation, anticipation, permission, and reinforcement
4. How to build the gradient in a classroom discussion and how to reestablish the environment when it has been violated in content, language, or style
5. How to achieve closure for a class or course

CREATING A SET

Educators often wonder how to begin a course or class. As a default, they begin with the housekeeping chores, which include any questions about the syllabus, room arrangements, class agreements, etc. Clearly, such a beginning does not enroll the learners to be excited about the course. Therefore all "housekeeping chores" can be delayed until after creation of the "set."

An effective "set" predisposes learners to be excited about the learning experience. It also opens the presentation and shapes the learning and attitudes of learners. Within this process a purpose for the course/class is created. An effective set:

- Captures the attention
- Engages the learners
- Motivates the participants to learn
- Promotes interest and attention to the topic
- Previews the class content and hints at what is to come
- Identifies objectives and expectations
- Creates anticipation

Notice that "telling a joke" is not in the above list. Unrelated humor can be used to begin a class, but it is more effective to begin with a question or story. The more traditional approach—telling the class what you will teach them, then teaching the content, and finally summarizing what you just taught them—is not an approach demonstrated in this chapter.

Example:

Prior to any discussion, housekeeping, roll call, or any other activity, hold up a nice ballpoint pen and ask the question, "Has this ever written a line of poetry?"

The response from learners may be silence, shuffling or quizzical expressions.

Simply wait until someone responds.

Some learners may respond positively or negatively.

Accept the negative response and follow up with the question, "What makes you say 'no'?"

Eventually someone will say, "Because people create poetry."

Then ask, "So what is the pen?"

At least a few learners will inform you that the pen is a "tool."

In reality, much of what is being taught in most courses is about tools. Such tools are very valuable, yet they are tools just the same. What is difficult for many educators is that the learners may choose to ignore these "valuable" tools and not use them. Or, if the educator has been successful in creating a positive, powerful learning environment, learners may take the tool set with them and consistently use it where appropriate. The learners are in **choice**. The challenge for the educator is to make the learning so powerful that learners want to use everything that is learned.

In thinking about this example, it becomes clear that the use of questions captures the attention of the learners; it clarifies at least one of the goals of the course, discovers the relevance of the learning for the course, and motivates the participant to learn.

The use of set, in a powerful way, creates the tone and the learning environment for the entire class or course. It is possible to create an overarching set for a course and then to create a mini-set for each of the classes in the course.

=== *FAST FACTS in a NUTSHELL*

- Begin each course and class with a "set."
- A set creates excitement for the learner about the course.

TOOLS THAT ENROLL THE LEARNER

Educators must acquire a set of tools and understanding to keep learners enrolled in the message. Basic concepts, such as the description of the average group of learners in the room, are a valuable beginning. In addition, specific strategies such as the use of anticipation are also valuable in keeping learners interested.

Class Composition

In any given class larger than 50, learners break down into four quadrants (see Exhibit 6.1). Quadrant #1 represents the learners who are extremely bright and the most difficult to keep engaged, the Quick Learners. They have captured the concept long before their classmates and are off thinking of something else while the educator is talking. Because we can think at a rate of more than 3,000 words per minute but only speak 300 words per minute, on average, this gap represents the time the quadrant #1 learners have to occupy their minds with something else. The effective educator utilizes tools discussed in this chapter to keep this group engaged.

Quadrant #4 learners (and there may not be many of these in nursing programs, or they may be the group for which English is a second language, or they may not be interested in the topic of the course) take a considerable amount of time to process the information and concepts. These are the Hard Workers. The challenge is to keep both quadrant #1 and quadrant #4 engaged regardless of the difference in their needs and abilities.

Quadrant #2 are excellent learners who usually sit in the front of the classroom and ask an abundance of questions. It

Exhibit 6.1   Distribution of Learners

Quadrant #1	Group 1: "Quick learners"
Quadrant #2	Group 2: "Processers"
Quadrant #3	Group 3: "Note takers"
Quadrant #4	Group 4: "Hard workers"

is easy for the educator to engage this group. Quadrant #3 learners sit more toward the middle of the classroom, take copious notes, and work hard. They can be quieter.

Experientially, the most resistant learners choose the back row beginning with the educator's back left hand side, and when that area is full, the other resistant learners choose the back right hand row. This information is helpful because the educator can surmise that if the back row is engaged, the entire classroom will be engaged.

================*FAST FACTS in a NUTSHELL*

- The GOAL is to engage the entire class.
- Understand the different levels of learning and engagement.

Anticipation

"This next tool is a learned skill. . . .

One I have to really concentrate on. . . .

It is a key concept in keeping all the learners in the room. . . .

It is also one of my favorite tools. . . ."

The dialogue above is an excellent example of how to create anticipation. Four comments were made, yet not one of them gave any structured information. When the educator creates anticipation, the quadrant #1 learners are attempting to discover what the point/content is that the educator is going to say. Their brains are overstimulated in the attempt to figure out what is coming next. At the same time quadrant #4 learners have time to move more slowly in the learning process.

Anticipation can be created by using the concept of known and unknown anticipation. Known anticipation is created when the educator announces that a quiz will begin each of the Monday class sessions. When teaching the content of this book in a workshop format, participants know that they will be video recorded each time they practice a new skill set in their small group. Great anxiety exists for learners who have never been video recorded. They enter class and see the video camera. This creates known anticipation and perhaps some anxiety.

Unknown anticipation is created when the statement or process is surprising. One example is the opening dialogue of this section; four statements were made and the learners had no idea what they meant or what would happen next in the classroom. Games or exercises in the classroom that are not preannounced create unknown anticipation. This anticipation keeps the learners guessing about what will come next and thus keeps them more engaged in the learning process.

═══════════════════════════════*FAST FACTS in a NUTSHELL*

- Develop strategies for keeping the learner engaged.
- Create both known and unknown anticipation.

Gradient

The rate at which something increases is known as gradient. The gradient can be increased gradually or rapidly. An example of gradually increasing the gradient can be understood in an initial nursing foundations course. An educator would not likely begin the first day of teaching the nursing process by discussing evaluation. That would be overgradient in relationship to content. Rather, the process begins with assessment, then development and implementation of the plan, and finally evaluation of the process. In other words, gradient implies developing a foundation and then building systematically until the most complex aspects of the process are reached.

The educator could be *overgradient* in terms of content, language, or style. In a discussion of disease processes, if the educator begins with a discussion of advanced physiology, the learners may appear stunned or blank. The educator is overgradient in terms of the content of the discussion. Likewise, if the educator uses a vocabulary in which every fourth word needs to be checked in the dictionary, this approach is overgradient in terms of language because the learners cannot understand the terminology or acronyms. Such discussions promote confusion rather than elucidation. Occasionally a few educators may use offensive language, such as swear words, which is also overgradient. A cardinal rule when teaching is to refrain at all times from using offensive language, because almost always at least one learner will be offended and this prohibits the active involvement of every learner in the classroom. Likewise, if the educator talks so fast that the learners cannot follow the presentation, their behavior constitutes being overgradient in terms of style. Other aspects of style that could be overgradient include having a superior attitude and speaking in a condescending fashion to the learners, or using very complex models that are unclear or convoluted.

The educator can also be *undergradient* in content, language, or style. This occurs when the educator attempts to provide basic content that everyone already knows. This is so boring that the learners will stop paying attention. Likewise, if the language used is at the 4th grade level, the learners may feel insulted. Or if the educator drones on in a style that clearly portrays a lack of interest in the topic, the style is undergradient.

Example:

What happens when the educator is overgradient in content?

The educator may say, "I'm seeing some blank faces. I believe I must have proceeded too rapidly. Let me try that again." And returning to where the educator believes she or he lost the learners, the educator begins to ask questions that help determine where the learners were lost. This is also known as seeking stable datum.

FAST FACTS in a NUTSHELL

- Observing the appropriate gradient honors the learner.
- Using the appropriate gradient supports learning in a gradual way.

Stable Datum

Stable datum is the point at which all learners in the room have the same knowledge base or experience. This is the point from which the educator can build and be sure that all the learners are either on the same page or starting the learning process from the same point. The educator simply asks questions until every hand is raised. It often helps to incorporate humor in this application.

Example:

"How many of you dissected a frog in high school biology?" Some hands will go up.

"Held a frog in your hand?" More hands will go up.

"Seen a frog?" More hands will go up.

"Seen a picture of a frog?" Now all the hands are raised. And people are chuckling.

Whatever anatomy or physiology point was to be made from dissection of a frog, at least everyone is now on equal footing and all have seen a frog.

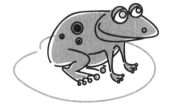

===============*FAST FACTS in a NUTSHELL*

- When the gradient is violated, always find stable datum.
- If the educator violates the gradient, apologize and establish stable datum.

Participation

Educators sometimes use a PowerPoint presentation as their notes and some may even read from the PowerPoint slides. According to Patricia Benner et al.'s (2010) most recent work, this is problematic for learning. Additionally, some educators even limit questions. Such behavior is counterintuitive to all the data we have about the effective ways in which adults learn. Adults learn through participation, discussion, and application of specific ideas and knowledge to how they will practice in the clinical area. If there is no focus on participation, educators could be replaced by a "talking head". To facilitate participation, some educators now provide an outline of the assigned reading and check the assignment at the classroom door. If the learner has not completed the outline, they are not admitted to the class. The expectation is that the learner will arrive at class having read the assignment and having begun to think about the application of this content. Class time is then devoted to application and synthesis of the knowledge from the assignment into how patients are cared for in the clinical setting. The extensive use of questions and such tools as positive reinforcement encourage learners in this process of thinking and clinical judgment as they apply to the practice of nursing. This translates to the educator needing to be knowledgeable about the many aspects of a clinical situation and able to lead a discussion of the situation using questions, positive reinforcement, clinical examples, and experience.

Example:

Teaching a class about Perinatal Loss and Bereavement might include chapters from *Association of Women's Health, Obstetrics and Neonatal Nursing's* (AWHONN's) perinatal textbook as well as the assigned text. When the learners arrive at class the discussion could focus on a couple of challenging scenarios and how the learners would provide care for the family in these difficult situations. Questions that encourage the use of the framework and possible interventions in the assigned literature could be explained and applied in the scenarios.

The scenarios could be debriefed after they are discussed to determine what was omitted. This would be a more successful approach than a PowerPoint presentation.

========================*FAST FACTS in a NUTSHELL*

- Adult learners apply knowledge through discussion.
- Expect learners to come to class prepared to discuss the learning works best.

Reinforcement/Acknowledgment

One tool that encourages participation is positive reinforcement or acknowledgment. In dialogue with learners, when the learner gives an appropriate or desired response, the educator must acknowledge it in a positive way. Reinforcement can be both verbal and non-verbal.

- Verbal reinforcement includes calling learners by their names, saying "Yes, great comment," repeating what was said, and comments such as "Tell me more, I like that thinking," "I agree," etc.
- Non-verbal reinforcement can be in the form of body language such as nodding the head in affirmation, using

hand gestures such as pointing to the person, or walking toward them. It includes writing what the learner said on a flip chart or giving a thumbs up, or a smile.

Positive reinforcement encourages dialogue in the classroom. Without it, learners are reticent to speak up or even to ask questions.

Educators do not always receive the correct answers and occasionally, learners are a bit fuzzy in their thinking. How are such situations handled?

The educator: "Thank you for that thought. . . . What do some of the rest of you think?"

Or, "Hummmm . . . Interesting. Can you tell me more about what makes you think that?"

Or, "Could you say more about your reasoning?"

Or, "What are the clinical ramifications of that solution?"

Notice that the educator did not say "no" or "you're wrong" or "not the right answer." Rather, the educator attempted to understand the thought process to be able to coach the learner and lead the learner through a process of discovery. This strategy leaves the learner with self-esteem intact, an interest in finding the answer, and an interest in learning. Of course, the goal is always to learn from any given situation.

When a complete acknowledgment is appropriate, specific guidelines for acknowledgment can make the situation very powerful (See Exhibit 1.2, p. 17). Attempt an acknowledgment of yourself using these guidelines.

FAST FACTS in a NUTSHELL

- You never learn less.
- Positive reinforcement makes the learner feel valued.

VARYING THE STIMULI

A key concept in keeping the learners enrolled is to vary the stimuli in the class. This can be accomplished in several ways, such as by using audiovisual enhancement and methods that stimulate the memory and by creating emotion. Creating emotions stimulates the limbic system and enhances long-term memory.

Accelerated Learning

The principles of accelerated learning stem from research done in the 1970s that sought to increase the ability of the human being to expand memory. This work stems from knowledge about the primary functions and where they are located in the brain. For example, the left brain focuses on vocabulary, numbers, and logic while the right brain focuses on creativity, music, and color (Rose & Nicholl, 1997).

When tools are used that seek to employ both sides simultaneously, the result is increased memory. Some educators now use music (the adagio movements of classical music, which is about 60 beats per minute) that coincides with the beating of the human heart. Color also enhances the ability to remember.

Visual Aids

Traditionally, *slides* or overhead transparencies were used to augment a lecture. Often, the educator used these as the outline for the content. In the worst cases, they were read; and they contained so many lines of material that it was impossible to see them from the back of the room. In addition, if learners were tired, they would take a nap because all the lights were turned off when the presentation began. This was not the best use of classroom time.

With the advent of technology, *PowerPoint presentations* were devised. The advantage of using PowerPoint was that the lights stayed on and it was harder for learners to nap. Otherwise, the same problems exist for PowerPoint that made slides difficult to use. *Overhead transparencies* functioned much the same way, except the educator could write on them during the presentation.

Some educators originally used blackboards and now may use whiteboards. At the same time some educators experimented with *flip charts*. This tool has the advantage of being used in the present. When they are posted around the classroom, they can be used to tie specific points together by walking over to an older one and connecting that content to the current point being made. They need to be in multiple colors so that both sides of the brain are engaged.

Video clips can be used to emphasize specific concepts. Many clips exist on YouTube. They can be serious or funny. For example, "Introducing Le Book" is a YouTube video that an educator might use to teach the concept of the human response to change. It is in Norwegian with subtitles and is staged in a monastery where the monks are changing from scrolls to bound books and having some difficulty. It is a parody of the current resistance to technological change. (Go to YouTube and find the clip, Introducing Le Book.)

Video clips from favorite movies are another audiovisual tool. For example, when teaching a course on powerful presentations, the educator can use clips from two movies that demonstrate excellent teaching strategies, "The Dead Poets Society" and "Mr. Holland's Opus." By choosing to view these films not for the story but for the creative methods of teaching, the educator will find a treasure trove.

Stories told by the educator are a wealth of information that can stimulate the memory. Many learners forget the content of a class but remember the poignant story. Many of these may be about patients and families. Most can be told, but some may be read. For example, a poem exists about giving up versus surviving.

Drowning or Surviving

Two frogs fell into a can of cream,
Or so I've heard it told.
The sides of the can were shiny and steep,
The cream was deep and cold,
"Oh, what's the use?" croaked No. 1,
"Tis fate; no help's around.
Goodbye, my friends! Goodbye, sad world!"
And weeping still, he drowned.

But No. 2, of sterner stuff,
Dog paddled in surprise,
The while he wiped his creamy face
And dried his creamy eyes.
"I'll swim awhile, at least," he said
Or so I've heard he said;
"It really wouldn't help the world
If one more frog were dead."

An hour or two he kicked and swam,
Not once he stopped to mutter,
But kicked and kicked and swam and kicked,
Then hopped out, via butter.

Anonymous

We all love stories of perseverance. After reading the story, the educator could pass out the story as a handout. Many educators have entire files, either paper or electronic, full of stories they have collected. These are a valuable resource.

Humor

The use of humor keeps learners engaged and stimulates discussion. It also helps to create relationships. Humor comes in the form of stories, jokes, or presentation style. For an educator to incorporate humor into the classroom, it is critically important to follow some simple rules:

1. *Never use humor that focuses on a minority or ethnic group.* Either someone or their best friend from that group will be in the room. This is particularly true of ethnic groups such as Polish Americans or groups such as physicians. The learner group can become very uncomfortable because they are thinking, "When will she poke fun at me or my group?" It is simply not worth the risk of disengaging the group.

2. *Use yourself as the brunt of humor or jokes.* Tell funny stories where the educator looked ridiculous or totally out of place. This conveys humanness and vulnerability and increases the opportunity that the learners will view the educator as a real, likable person.

Stories and humor are such an important part of the educator's tool bag that an entire chapter has been devoted to the subject. (See Chapter 9, Telling Stories)

Experiential Learning

Experiential learning is a powerful adult learning tool that allows the learner to practice the professional role or to learn a concept in a different way.

Examples:

Exercises: When attempting to teach a concept, the educator can use a brief exercise. If an educator was attempting to clarify both the concept of multitasking (very popular at this time!) and the research that suggests that multitasking is not necessarily positive, the educator could ask for a volunteer learner and do the following:

1. Count from one to ten as quickly as possible.

2. Say the "a,b,c's" as quickly as possible.

3. Finally put the two tasks together as in 1,a, 2,b, 3,c, 4,d, 5,e, etc.

If the educator is timing each event, the demonstration will take about 4–7 seconds to accomplish the first two tasks and more than 20 seconds to accomplish the last task. Often all the learners will laugh and then the debrief can follow.

Games: With the advent of the Internet, an abundance of games is available to accomplish many different objectives. For example, if the educator is discussing the concept of *change* and wants to demonstrate through playing the Change Game, he might have the group break into dyads:

1. They face each other and study each other very carefully as to what they look like or are wearing.

2. Turn back-to-back for 30 seconds and each changes five things about their own appearance.

3. Turn to face their own partners again and identify the things that have been changed. Many people feel stretched to change five things about their appearance, which may be indicative of how they feel about change in general.

4. Next have them turn back-to-back again and change an additional seven things about their appearance. They cannot change anything back to the way it was originally, but they may change something a second time. Much distress is the norm.

5. Then have them turn face-to-face and identify the changes each other made.

6. The third time, they turn back-to-back and change another five things about their appearance. Full-blown groaning probably ensues. In the debrief, it is

important for the entire room to notice what people have changed: Did they only take things off or did they also add things to their appearance? It provides a real sense of how different people adapt to change.

Small groups/dyads: When learners are practicing a specific skill set, dyads can be very helpful. For example, if educators are teaching coaching as a skill set, each learner in the room would want to practice these skills. These dyads can be established so that each learner has an opportunity to play each role. Then a general debrief is helpful.

Role Playing: When teaching how to deal with difficult questions or upset people, the educators can role play the initial example for the learners. The role play can be scripted, but they are often more fun when they are done extemporaneously by the educators. They are often funny and the educators can look inadequate or stumped. The learners love when the educators make mistakes just like they do.

Simulations: Simulations can range from minimal use of simulators to a full cardiac arrest simulation using a $200,000 mannequin that can be intubated, resuscitated, etc. Many scenarios have been created that help teach learners. And videotaping the simulation is very powerful. The crucial element of any simulation is the debriefing (which will be discussed in Chapter 12).

Even with this brief discussion of experiential learning, it becomes clear how powerful this tool is and how important it is to integrate the classroom time with this type of learning.

FAST FACTS in a NUTSHELL

- Stories and humor promote engagement and memory.
- Use exercises, games, small groups, and experiential learning.

PERMISSION

To build trust and to role model professional behavior, it is important for the educator to work with learners in ways that honor them as human beings and future professionals. If the educator doesn't treat the learners honorably, how can they be expected to treat each other or patients and their families honorably? This translates into refusing to put the learners "on the spot" by randomly calling on them to respond to the educator's questions. Rather, the educator can ask such questions as "If you would be willing . . .?" or "Who can tell me . . .?" If the learner group is nonresponsive, another strategy is to tell the learners at the beginning of class that today the expectation will be for the learners to respond to questions in order around the circle or down the row. This provides a warning at the beginning that learners can expect to be "called upon" to respond to questions.

=====*FAST FACTS in a NUTSHELL*

- Honoring learners is a demonstration of how to treat other human beings.

CLOSURE

The ending of the class or the course should not be "Well, I see we are out of time. . . ." or "Are there any questions?" Questions should be next to last. The closing must find a way to connect the content and new learning to what was already known or how the learner should use the new information or processes in the practice of nursing.

- The educator can ask the learners how they will use the class content to further their goals or objectives. This process can help the learners in their attempt to apply and synthesize learning.

- The educator could also use a story, poem, or video clip that illustrates a major point from the class. An important aspect of closure is to engage the limbic system of the learner through some type of emotion. The emotion imprints the story, poem, clip, etc. so that it can be remembered. In this way the learning is connected to an emotion and it is more easily remembered.

Example:

When teaching communication and active listening (which is something many of us have difficulty with), ending the class by reading a poem such as that in Exhibit 6.1, emphasizes in a memorable way how important listening is for human beings.

═══════════════*FAST FACTS in a NUTSHELL*

- Memorable closings solidify learning.
- Connecting class content and previous knowledge enhances learning.

Exhibit 6.1   Poem, "Listen"

When I ask you to listen to me
And you start giving me advice,
You have not done what I asked.

(continued)

Exhibit 6.1 (*continued*)

When I ask you to listen to me
And you begin to tell me 'why' I shouldn't
    feel that way,
You are trampling on my feelings.

When I ask you to listen to me
And you feel you have to do something to
    solve my problems,
You have failed me, strange as that may seem.

Listen! All I ask is that you listen;
Not talk, nor do—just hear me.

And I can do for myself—I'm not helpless
Maybe discouraged and faltering, but not helpless.

When you do something for me, that I can
    and need to do for myself,
You contribute to my fear and weakness.

But when you accept as a simple fact that I do feel
    what I feel,
No matter how irrational
Then I quit trying to convince you
And can get about the business of understanding
What's behind this irrational feeling.

When that's clear,
The answers are obvious and I don't need advice.

(*continued*)

Exhibit 6.1   *(continued)*

Irrational feelings make sense when we
    understand what's behind them.

Perhaps that's why prayer works sometimes for
    some people;
because God is mute, and doesn't give
    advice to try to 'fix' things,
He/She just listens, and lets you work it out
    for yourself.

So please listen, and just hear me, and if you
    want to talk,
Wait a minute for your turn,
And I'll listen to you.

Anonymous

*This poem was written by a mental health consumer
who was institutionalized over a number of years in
Queensland. He wishes to remain anonymous.*

SYNTHESIS

Using these concepts supports the engagement of the learners in the topic that the educator is teaching. Permission and
positive reinforcement encourage learners to participate in
classroom activities. Creating a set at the beginning of a class
helps learners understand the purpose of the class. Closure
for the class supports learners to understand and integrate
the purpose of the class. Skillful educators use all these tools
to increase the likelihood that learners will be engaged in the
learning process and apply the knowledge learned.

7

Coaching Learners

*Learners are our future. It is up to us as the coaches,
the guides, the educators to instill the importance
of the message. The educator is "sitting in practice"
and the coaching provided about care is the best
possible learning we can provide.*

Lori Rodriguez, PhD, RN

INTRODUCTION

*Coaching is an important strategy to use with all learners,
especially with those who may be reluctant to actively
participate and those who may be exceptional learners.
It could be seen as the ultimate "use of self" to facilitate learning. Coaching is designed to help the recipients of the process discover for themselves answers that
can help in future situations. It can be used in individual
situations as well as in the classroom with a group of
learners participating. It builds on who the person is
rather than focusing on specific behaviors or ways of
acting that are deemed as "the right way." This strategy
capitalizes on the strength of reflection and has international applicability.*

In this chapter, you will learn:

1. What coaching is
2. How to use coaching effectively
3. How to communicate clearly
4. How to give feedback
5. How to coach for performance
6. How to coach in the classroom

WHAT COACHING IS

The International Coach Federation (n.d.) defines coaching as "a thought-provoking and creative process that inspires them [the recipient of the process] to maximize their personal and professional potential." Thus, coaching enables the educator to encourage learners to grow through a positive interaction. In short, coaches attempt to build an individual's strengths through a process that supports individual insight. Williamson, in Donner and Wheeler (2009), refers to the coach as the midwife who supports and guides an individual through a process. Coaching is so important that Benner et al. (2010) suggest that educators need to learn how to coach.

Unlike mentoring, which typically involves a longer term relationship between someone with more experience and someone with less, coaching is a collaboration between someone who has the ability to coach and someone who is willing to engage in the coaching process to attain goals.

Some coaching can occur in the classroom, and the wise educator will use coaching in other settings when working with individual learners.

- In the classroom, coaching might be used to move a learner to a deeper or broader thinking or to the "better" answer.
- In individual situations, more specifics (such as poor performance or apparent boredom) can be explored from the learner's perspective.

Coaching can help the coach gain insight into the rationale behind specific answers or actions. In doing so, if the learner has fully engaged in the coaching session, the learner gains self-insight that can be used in future situations to improve performance.

═══════════════════*FAST FACTS in a NUTSHELL*

- Coaching is an interactive process designed to build on strengths.
- Coaching focuses on helping the learner to develop self-insight.
- The art of coaching is analogous to the art of midwifery.

HOW TO USE COACHING EFFECTIVELY

1. *Professional Relationship*—Coaching creates a more intimate relationship with a learner because the educator is "seeing" how the learner thinks. The professional relationship, where the goal is to help the learner be more effective in learning, is the focus of coaching. Coaching is not designed to become a therapeutic or exploratory relationship. Thus, educators need to consider carefully with whom to engage in a coaching situation and to be explicit about the nature of coaching.
2. *Mutuality*—The coaching process relies on mutuality. The recipient (learner) must have the trust and appreciation of the coach and the coach must have the trust and appreciation of the recipient (learner). Without that mutuality, the full benefit of coaching cannot be achieved. Additionally, each individual must respect the other and believe that the shared coaching experience is mutually beneficial. The learner benefits in terms of self-insight and the coach

benefits from helping each learner with whom this strategy is employed to become more self-reliant and confident. Trust, appreciation, and respect are not something gained automatically because one person is an educator and the other is a learner. All three are earned. Thus, individual coaching is not an initial strategy.

3. *Communication and Self-Discovery*—One of the key strategies in coaching is to ask questions that lead the learner to self-discovery. Chapter 8 discusses the topic of questions and some of those apply to coaching. Subsequent sections in this chapter describe the coaching communication process and include some questions.

4. *Agreement on Anticipated Outcome*—Two other strategies employed are to agree to what the anticipated outcome might be and to what will occur. These two strategies are typically used in out-of-class coaching activities. In the classroom, however, educators can use class agreements and state what the anticipated outcome might be. Chapter 4 describes agreements. Anticipated outcomes should relate to the curriculum, course, or module objectives as well as to the learners' needs.

5. *Agreement on What Will Occur*—In individual coaching efforts, agreeing to what will occur entails creating the details. These details might involve addressing the following questions:

   • What questions will the learner bring?
   • How often would a "regular session" be scheduled and how long should each last?
   • Does a specific question/issue need to be evident to the learner to precipitate a session?
   • Will the setting be formal or not?
   • Can coaching occur via phone or the Internet?

   These kinds of agreements, discussed early in a relationship with a learner, set the limits of what will be effective for the learner and the educator. This same discussion can be held at the beginning of a course so that learners know what to expect in the classroom.

6. *Coaching That Has a Specific Goal*—Coaching might be specific and thus the anticipated outcome is specific. For example, for the learner who isn't doing well in class but has performed satisfactorily in the past, the anticipated outcome might be to explore what the positive in-class performance looked like, what its relevance to the learner was, and how that "picture" differs from the current reality.

7. *Coaching That Is More Broadly Based*—Coaching also might be more broadly based and thus the outcome may be stated in broader terms. For example, for the learner who quickly grasps content and is ready to move to another topic more rapidly than others in a group, the learner may identify the issue as one of boredom. The anticipated outcome might also be broad: to feel more engaged, to be less bored, to gain self-insight, etc.

While learners may come with these broad goals, an educator who uses coaching effectively can use the coaching process to get to a clearly defined issue and a clearly defined outcome. For example, if the learner (above) is bored, documenting how boredom manifests itself and then creating a plan to increase the time of engagement (for example, thinking about how learners learn) might be helpful.

═══════════════════════════*FAST FACTS in a NUTSHELL*

- Mutuality is a critical element of a positive, effective coaching situation.
- Making anticipated outcomes clear improves the coaching experience.

HOW TO COMMUNICATE CLEARLY

In order for a coach, or an educator, to be effective, the learner or learners need to perceive that the coach or educator truly cares about their success as learners.

1. The first step in communicating clearly as a coach is to listen intensely. Hearing what the learner is saying often provides insight to the educator about what to probe that will best produce insight for the learner. Listening for specific words, tonality, volume, and so forth are all clues upon which the coach may act. Thus, shutting out (literally and figuratively) the external noises is critical. As in any good communication exchange, if you aren't clear what the person is saying, paraphrase what was said to see if the person agrees that was the message.

2. The questions related to coaching are designed to have the learner say more about the topic, to expand on any statements in a reflective manner, and to learn from the process. As an example, the coach and learner may engage in a conversation that looks like this:

   Learner: I am feeling anxious that I don't know enough despite the *As* I have earned on the tests.

   Coach: Tell me more.

   Learner: Well, I see these thick textbooks and I see how many websites are devoted to a disease and then I do a literature search and I find hundreds of articles in the past five years. If I can't be the best nurse, I don't want to be one.

   Coach: When you think about the "best nurse," what are the behaviors the best nurse demonstrates?

   This conversation conveys that the learner is doing well and yet feels overwhelmed by the amount not yet studied. The question the educator raises in the end precipitates the opportunity to consider the relationship between studying and reading and being the best nurse.

3. Emphasize the use of open-ended questions. Note that the questions and statements in the example are phrased as open-ended ones. Although an educator may use close-ended questions to validate information (for example, "Did that make sense?"), the emphasis has to be on open-ended questions to stimulate self-reflection. Exhibit 7.1 presents examples of key open-ended questions/statements to use in coaching situations.

Exhibit 7.1 Questions/Statements for Coaching

How did you feel when then happened?

How does this fit with your goal?

Please elaborate.

What more would you add?

When you did that, what were you thinking about?

If you were faced with the situation again, what would you do to facilitate an outcome more in alignment with what you desire?

How was that action typical of you?

What would happen if…?

Please describe another situation where this approach (something discussed) would work.

════════════════*FAST FACTS in a NUTSHELL*

- Begin with listening intently.
- Paraphrase for clarity.
- Use open-ended questions to stimulate the learner to "find" the answers.
- Use close-ended questions when seeking validation.

HOW TO GIVE FEEDBACK

In addition to communicating clearly through questions and explorations, coaches provide feedback.

1. Feedback is designed to provide honest observations. These observations may be about the whole event (for example, "I sense you are making progress in reaching your goal of trying to balance your home life with your school life") or about some specific element (for example, "I noted that you smiled when you said what you really thought of that assignment").

2. Feedback is also designed to help learners reach greater understanding through validation from others. For example, the insecure learner needs to hear validation from the educator. In this example, it would also be important to explore how the learner feels when validated and to determine what signs the learner can find individually so that the coach eventually is no longer needed.

3. Specific feedback is more useful in helping to shape the learner's behavior. Rather than saying something such as "You are doing a great job of meeting your goal," consider something that is specific, and preferably recent—for example, "Your statement about not wanting to miss any lectures even when you are sick was useful in understanding your rationale for not complying with the illness policy." This example could launch a bigger discussion about why the illness policy is in place.

4. Feedback also must be honest. If it is clear that the learner didn't think deeply on a topic, saying something to the contrary causes the learner to mistrust the coaching activity. That is really the whole point of coaching for learning: to stimulate deeper thinking that helps learners filter out less important information and focus on that which is important.

Journaling

One method of providing feedback is to agree to use a journal as a communication device. The learner records anything in the journal that pertains to the agreed-upon coaching focus. The educator can provide comments throughout (either electronically or in a hand-written format) in order to cause the learner to think more on some aspect of an entry.

Journaling is a process used by many people. Some people use it as therapy, recording various feelings and concerns. Other people are required to keep them for historical purposes, such as the British royalty. Here the purpose of a journal relates to the educator helping the learner gain self-insight. Thus this type of journal is, in a sense, a reflection of the learner's professional development (see pp. 22–23). It can reflect facts, attitudes, insights, and so forth regarding the topic of discussion. To achieve the expectations for this type of journal, learners will need to think critically and creatively.

Exhibit 7.2 depicts an example of an interchange in a journal. Note that the educator has used the underline feature rather than the track changes function. Logically, an educator would not ask all of those questions after each statement. However, any of the examples could help learners see

---

Exhibit 7.2   Journal Interchange

After Mr. J returned from the PACU, I immediately checked his orders and then him. <u>How did his arrival change the care for your other patients? Clarification: Was the above the sequence of your activity? What would happen if you first checked him and then the orders? How did you determine if your findings were appropriate for someone just returning to his primary unit?</u>*

*Underlined words represent the educator's feedback.

different perspectives on their behavior. Having the learners return their comments in the subsequent time period allows the educator to see what the learner has done with the prior feedback and thus how to proceed with the next.

=== *FAST FACTS in a NUTSHELL*

- Being as specific as possible helps the learner to validate and learn what is important.
- Journaling provides a written approach to coaching.

HOW TO COACH FOR PERFORMANCE

One of the most important aspects of coaching is to match the level of the content and the level of the learner(s) in relation to the content and objectives. Starting at basic levels for beginning learners is logical. However, the coaching activity shouldn't be designed to "reteach" the knowledge, skills, and attitudes of the learner.

One strategy to use at all levels is to match the desired objective. This strategy assumes some type of preparation was expected prior to the classroom engagement. If learners are struggling with solid responses, pause and ask a question such as one of those found in Exhibit 7.3. These questions are designed to help learners recall what they know that is relevant to the current discussion.

Exhibit 7.3 Questions Designed to Match Objectives

What can be recalled from the pathophysiology of this condition?

(continued)

Exhibit 7.3 *(continued)*

In X course, you learned about the importance of understanding what it means to assume leadership in clinical situations. What are some examples of assuming leadership here?

Even if you didn't know anything about the medication, how would you determine if it was safe to administer it to someone on coumadin therapy?

If you were in a community setting and the patient suddenly revealed another, a previously unknown, diagnosis, what process would you use to determine the importance of this condition?

Think back to your nutrition course. Now consider this: In a household of obese children, how can you help the primary caregiver understand what nutrition is and how it influences health?

FAST FACTS in a NUTSHELL

- Relate the coaching feedback to specific, desired outcomes.
- Start where learners should be and use a recall technique if such is warranted.

HOW TO COACH IN THE CLASSROOM

Unlike individual coaching sessions where only the educator and learner are present, coaching in the classroom has many observers. The probing questions used during an open session such as a classroom would need to focus on content, process, and outcomes rather than personal perspectives.

An exception to this might be found when the content is controversial (for example, creating public policy or an ethical decision). While the personal perspective may be challenged, the person, as such, should not be. An example of this point follows:

> *Educator:* Let's assume that Tim's point is the best view and remember, there are many legislators and a good percentage of the public who agree. If you were in opposition, how could you diminish the importance of this view?
>
> *Learner 1:* I'd just tell Tim he didn't have a grip on reality!
>
> *Educator:* That is exactly how some people would respond. Let's explore where that takes us in diminishing the importance of the view Tim provided.

Note that the educator acknowledged the assumptions; acknowledged the reality that no matter what someone says, a group of people with similar views exists; and that rather than discounting a response that sounds as if it is a beginning of an argument, the educator again acknowledged the statement as a view of some people. The educator is focusing on the content of the perspective, not the person who voiced the perspective.

Setting the expectation about the role of the observers during an open coaching session not only keeps all learners engaged but also provides them with an important role to fill.

- For example, an educator may choose to have only one learner engaged in responses. In that case, the educator can ask the other learners to write key words in response to the questions and then hold a more open discussion at the end of the observation period.
- In another example, asking what someone recorded when questioned about what a particular disease process interrupted in normal physiological functioning could create the opportunity to see how multiple events unfold from a pathological condition. Some learners might want to describe the precise mechanism at the cellular

level for what is transpiring, whereas someone else may have a one-word response. This discussion opens up for all the opportunity to see how differently we learn and how we can learn from each other. The educator may also encourage the group to respond. In that case, finding the "best answer" and then deciding what made it "best" might help learners discover words, phrases, or concepts that link important knowledge to a given situation. This sharing helps learners see how to evaluate responses to get to the "best answer" and to see how others view situations.

Meaningful coaching resides in facilitating the birthing process (to use the midwifery analogy) of new perspectives about a situation. Thus, declaring that "We are now going to walk through the coaching process" is ineffective. When learners are sending signals that some concept is escaping them, pause, back up to the prior point, and ask a question. If someone responds with a good or "best" answer, use that statement to further explore the concept so that the key related elements are discussed. Then—and this is especially helpful—summarize the key elements so that everyone is sure what they were. The difference in coaching (or, as the next chapter discusses, in asking questions) to the best response is that the learners are actively engaged in thinking through the situation or concept in order to participate in the discussion and get to the "best answer" themselves.

═══════*FAST FACTS in a NUTSHELL*

- Engage learners even if they aren't responding orally to questions.
- Focus on moving learners to the best response.
- Focus on exploring the rationale behind the best response.

SYNTHESIS

Coaching individuals and groups helps them to find their own answers. This approach better prepares new graduates for the real world of practice where they may have to be somewhat self-reliant. Coaching involves a structured approach of alerting learners about what is going to happen and then working with them to gain self-insight. The intent is always to move learners to intense thinking and reflection.

8

Asking Questions

An inquisitive nurse educator guides, directs, and cultivates inquiry through insightful questions. It's not the answer but the question that sustains creative and critical inquiry!

Donna M. Nickitas, PhD, RN, NEA-BC, CNE

INTRODUCTION

Asking questions is a highly effective strategy to engage learners, assess what learners know, and support clinical thinking. Knowing when and how to ask questions is critical to being effective as a facilitator of learning. Questions aren't always presented in the form of a question; rather, an actual statement (e.g., "Tell me more") can produce the same effect of engaging learners in actively participating in a conversation that is directed through them rather than merely presented to them.

In this chapter, you will learn:

1. Why to ask questions
2. What questions to ask

3. When to ask questions
4. How to word effective questions
5. Who asks questions

WHY ASK QUESTIONS?

Asking questions is a time-consuming task that requires pre-planning. This doesn't mean that as a conversation unfolds other questions might not come to mind. Rather, it means that effective teaching requires educators to determine what is important for learners to know as well as to determine what questions will help learners analyze, synthesize, apply, and evaluate their current knowledge in considering the care of patients and populations.

- Asking questions helps educators determine what a learner or group of learners recall and how they proceed to think through situations to arrive at a desired answer.
- Asking questions requires that learners remain engaged in the process to follow the unfolding information that allows them to discover the desired outcomes.

Educators serve as facilitators for helping learners pull from their own reservoirs of knowledge and also serve as augmenters of that knowledge as needed. This is in contrast to a frequently used more "secure" approach of "filling the hour" with content so that no questions could be asked that might not be easily answered. This passive approach, often referred to as straight lecturing, puts the educators in charge of being accountable for all that learners need to know, and it often loses learners intellectually because their individual thinking processes aren't in harmony with that of the educator who is presenting. Exhibit 8.1 (p. 118) reflects common purposes of questions.

Questions can be convergent, a pulling together, or divergent, a dispersion. Convergent questions typically form the "best approach" or synthesis responses. An example of a convergent question would be: "From all that we looked at today, what can we conclude about Jason and his family?" Another example would be: "Based on our consideration of various nursing strategies, what would be our best approach in providing care for Mr. Astonophos?" Divergent questions are designed to create options. The simplest form of a divergent question is "What else?"

In practice, an educator might ask divergent questions to stimulate possibilities and then follow that with convergent questions to create the best approach from among those presented. The wise educator is always prepared with other questions if a true lag in responses occurs. As an example, the educator might ask, "Do you think massage would be useful?" Someone responds affirmatively and the educator follows with another question such as, "What makes you say 'yes'?" The greatest error educators can make relative to questions (other than not asking them at all!) is to ask, "Are there any questions?" pause for a second, and then continue talking. Silence helps learners formulate questions, gather courage to ask a question, and synthesize what was discussed. Having a true pause conveys that the educator truly values questions from the learners.

═══════════════*FAST FACTS in a NUTSHELL*

- Asking questions engages the learner in the learning process.
- Asking questions requires preplanning the questions so they facilitate learning.
- Asking questions can help educators assess learners' knowledge and clinical thinking processes.

WHAT QUESTIONS NEED TO BE ASKED?

Several sources influence what questions to ask. Some obvious ones are the course objectives; evidence-based care, licensure, or certification examinations; and critical or common care requirements. Less obvious ones include expectations of prospective employers, the latest research related to content previously studied, and the distinctive considerations of a particular patient-care situation. Content is driven by course or module objectives. Those elements of the curriculum also convey the expected level of attainment of knowledge, skills, and attitudes. A common form of domain classifications across the curriculum would be useful to educators as they try to match the outcomes for the new graduate. (If a common form of domain classifications is unavailable, consider the information found at www.projects.coe.uga.edu/epltt/index .php?title=Bloom%27s_Taxonomy)

Because the focus at most levels of professional education is on the application, synthesis, and valuing of knowledge, that is where questions need to be directed. As an example, although an educator might need to ask a recall-type question ("How does norepinephrine work?"), the real focus should be on higher level cognitive activities such as those that might be present in a case study. The educator might ask questions such as: "What would you anticipate as a complication for this patient?" and "How would you plan for that?" Looking at the higher level cognitive objectives helps learners to be better prepared for clinical situations and enhances their potential for being successful on standardized tests.

Because nursing's strength is found in nurses' clinical reasoning abilities, rote learning and recall questions do little to facilitate this development. Even when teaching nonclinical subjects (e.g., content that includes history) it is important to determine what learners know about what was happening in health care, society, and the world as the context for considering why nurses took a specific action. If learners don't know the answers to such questions, ask a question such as: "How do you think you will be able to find that information before we consider this topic again?" Obviously if the educator wants learners to seek the information, that expectation needs to be formally stated.

════════════════════FAST FACTS in a NUTSHELL

- Questions focused on higher level cognitive objectives are more useful in facilitating learning than are questions focused on lower level objectives.
- Educators may need to return to lower level cognitive objectives if learners struggle with higher level ones.
- Using strategies that promote questions (such as case studies) helps learners actively engage in learning and helps them think through the situation.

WHEN IS THE TIME TO ASK QUESTIONS?

Starting a learning session with the expectation that learners have completed assignments prior to arriving allows an educator to move directly to questions that promote learning and reinforce what learners have read. Although questions can be asked at any point in the class session, asking them early in an interaction engages learners in the learning process. These questions (such as those used thus far in this chapter) can organize content that might need to be presented if learners are inaccurate in their responses or if they don't participate (although that behavior poses other issues discussed elsewhere). If higher level objectives–based questions cannot be answered readily, moving to lower level objectives–based questions can facilitate learning. Additionally, an educator may choose to start with lower level questions and then continue to build on the responses to lead learners to higher level thinking. If this approach is used, moving quickly to high-level questions will simulate the clinical experience. Because the normal attention span of adults is about 20 minutes (Dukette & Cornish, 2009), asking questions one or more times during that time interval keeps learners engaged in learning.

Other factors to consider related to timing include the following:

- Call the learners back to a key focus of a learning session.
- Test if learners are grasping content of a discussion or reading assignment.
- Reengage learners with each other in the process of learning.

One well-documented approach is derived from the Harvard Assessment Seminars (Light, 1986), which reported several strategies to enhance college teaching. Among those strategies was the use of the "one-minute paper":

- At the end of the class period, the faculty member asks learners to take out a piece of paper (which is probably the best technique today to allow for anonymity, even though learners could email or text responses before leaving the room).
- Two questions are posed that literally are to be answered in no more than 1 minute each. The questions are: "What was the big idea you learned in class today?" and "What was the unclear point from the class today?" (Light, 1986, p. 3.7). (This approach is discussed in greater detail in Chapter 11, Seeking Input.) Those questions can be varied, for example, by asking, "What was the big point today and what questions remain?"

- Prior to the next class session, the faculty member reviews those items and uses them as the reinforcing points and questions to review.
- Another strategy is to provide a synopsis of the two questions in, for example, the online portion of a course, so that all learners can see what others saw as the big points and what questions others had.

═══════════════════════════*FAST FACTS in a NUTSHELL*

- Starting questions early in a class session sets the tone and engages learners.
- Focus on high-level questions to replicate the situations learners find in their clinical experiences.
- Use a strategy such as the "Big Point/What Questions Remain?" approach to validate where learners are in their grasp of complex content.

HOW SHOULD QUESTIONS BE PHRASED TO BE EFFECTIVE?

The answer to how questions need to be phrased is equally as important as any of the other elements related to the basics of questions. Asking questions that can be answered with simple answers such as "yes" or "no" promote little learning. Anyone answering that type of question has a 50% chance of answering correctly. Unless there are obvious signs of guessing (e.g., saying the answer in a manner that sounds as if it is another question), an educator would not know if the learner answered based on knowledge or based on luck. However, asking yes/no questions can be effective if they are accompanied with the statement, "Provide your rationale for your answer."

Exhibit 8.1 provides several examples of how to word questions. First, note there are no "why" questions. Educators can ask questions that get to the "why" of a situation without ever using that word. For example, rather than asking why someone answered as he or she did, educators could ask what the rationale was in reaching a particular conclusion, as presented above. Second, note that none of the examples in Exhibit 8.1 can be answered in a simplistic manner, except for the one related to validating understanding. This means that learners have to process data and knowledge to make conclusions. Third, various questions serve different purposes. The more generic the question, the more useful it is across the curriculum. For example, the question: "How do you see what happened here?" might serve many purposes. It could be equally applicable in the classroom and clinical settings, at an entry level course or in the final semester, or for physiological or behavioral issues.

Exhibit 8.1   Examples of Questions by Purpose

Purpose of Question	Example
Persuade others	What would prevent you from saying yes to this agreement?
Gain information	How do you see what happened here?
Plant your own ideas	So, if we implement the idea you just offered, and this other idea (which I offered), what do you think the outcome might be?
Clarify vague answers	What are the steps you would use to make that work?

(continued)

Exhibit 8.1 (*continued*)

Purpose of Question	Example
Motivate others	How do you think others would see this solution meeting their needs?
Solve problems	How would it work to implement your idea?
Soften criticism	How do you think others react when your part of the project isn't done on time?
Hear another view	From what perspective do you think pharmacists see this issue?
Validate understanding	Can you summarize your plan to complete this assignment? (Note this question is a forced choice yes/no question that needs further follow up, such as "Great! What is the plan?" [if the answer was yes], or "I'm concerned that you have no plan. How will you proceed?" [if the answer was no].)
Overcome objections	What are the major concerns you have with moving ahead with this plan?
Refocus attention	How does that point relate to the key discussion?
Redirecting the question	How might we answer Tom's question?

(*continued*)

Exhibit 8.1 *(continued)*

Purpose of Question	Example
Gain cooperation	What would prevent you from saying yes to this agreement? (Note that this is essentially the same question used to persuade. The same question can serve multiple purposes.)
Reduce anxiety	How does this approach make you feel?
Defuse volatile situations	Could you give me an example of what was so frustrating?
Gain control	How do you see your performance in relation to the criteria/objectives?
Think futuristically	Based on the rapid advances in sciences affecting nursing, what will practice be like in 5 years?

Based on Kowalski, K. (2009a). More situations in which questions are valuable. *The Journal of Continuing Education in Nursing: Continuing Competence for the Future, 40*(9), 393; and Kowalski, K. (2009b). Situations in which questions are valuable. *The Journal of Continuing Education in Nursing: Continuing Competence for the Future, 40*(8), 344–345.

FAST FACTS in a NUTSHELL

- The format for a question should require a sentence or more as a response.
- Creating a finely honed question in a generic format can be used for multiple purposes.

WHO ASKS QUESTIONS

Many educators have had the experience in which educators ask questions and learners respond. In other instances, educators may have talked for the majority of the time and then "left time for questions." Learning can be facilitated by helping learners know that they too need to ask questions and participate throughout the time together. In other words, questions are formed to create the dialogue that occurs related to a condition or topic. This exchange of questions allows both learners and educators to direct the nature of the learning. While that may seem a little frightening because not all of the content was covered, it is equally scary to consider that learners and educators spent a designated amount of time together and neither understood where the other was in their thinking. If we are to create clinical reasoning, as Benner et al. (2010) suggested, the focused dialogues, enriched by questions, provide for high-level knowledge development.

When learners ask questions, paraphrasing the question not only reflects your attentiveness but also allows for clarification of the question. For example, if a question is complex, the educator might say: "So, I hear three questions. First, is . . ." If the educator chooses not to answer a particular question, a good strategy is redirection by asking, "What responses do you all have for this question?" The dialogue that ensues can further be supported by asking for the evidence that supports the responses provided.

SYNTHESIS

To be effective, educators could consider writing out core questions, such as the examples discussed above. Practicing—even with colleagues—can help break the habit of answering questions automatically. Oral questions should be as well thought out as written questions. They need to be clear and positively stated to avoid confusion on the responder's part. When negative questions are used, learners can become confused about whether they are answering the core question or the "not" part. For example, asking, "What would you expect to find if you suspected abuse?" (a positively state question) is clearer for learners than asking: "What wouldn't you expect to find if you suspected abuse?" (a negatively stated question).

If educators have large numbers of learners in a setting, several options exist for using questions. For example, after dividing the learners into groups, it is possible to ask the same question(s) of each group. Alternatively, it might be preferable to use a common learning tool (such as a case study), and then provide different questions to different groups. If the latter strategy is used, bringing smaller groups together to gain insight into the bigger perspective will be helpful. Additionally, it is possible, if the questions are very focused, to have serial discussions. For example, Group 1 might be asked to determine what the main concern of the patient is. That conclusion is reported to Group 2, who can either accept the finding or challenge it and then answer the next question (e.g., how to decide what to do). Group 3 could be asked to determine what clinical measures might be used to determine if the prior discussions were effective, and so forth.

Focusing the class session around questions rather than objectives helps learners know they are expected to engage in some dialogue rather than merely listen. Guiding learners through questions further supports their clinical learning opportunities because the same kinds of questions can be used to reason through patient care situations.

9

Telling Stories

Telling stories about yourself and your professional development is a popular teaching strategy. I tell stories I think carry a message, for example ones in which I made a mistake or ones in which I am the heroine, or ones in which I get my comeuppance. Those stories teach accountability, professional insight and humility, respectively. The most vivid are those in which I fail at the professional task, but triumph in my insight and commitment to new learning. If such stories are told with passion and integrity, I have found that learners remember the story, and more importantly the moral of the story, many years later.

Eileen Zungolo, EdD, RN, ANEF

INTRODUCTION

Keeping learners engaged in the learning process is a key part of being an effective educator. One of the most highly effective strategies is telling stories, if the story is told in a dynamic manner so that learners are motivated to listen carefully for clues as to what happens next. The point of a story is to "paint a picture" of a patient, clinical situation, or professional issue so that the learner feels transported into the story itself.

In this chapter, you will learn:

1. What storytelling is
2. What the key elements of a story are
3. How to construct a story to maintain learners' interest
4. When to use stories in the classroom
5. What to expect of learners as a result of their hearing a story

WHAT IS STORYTELLING?

Storytelling is a deliberate form of communication designed to help others learn. Storytelling has specific elements, all of which are designed to heighten the listeners' attention. Almost everyone has some exposure to stories. Children often are tucked into bed with the ritualistic practice of a parent or older sibling reading a story. Grandparents and elders in the community often tell stories about how things were some number of years back. Native American culture, among others, is passed on through the sacred tradition of sharing messages from the past with the younger members of the tribes. Storyteller dolls show a person surrounded by children crawling all over, because stories attract. A well-constructed story allows an educator to engage knowledge, skills, and attitudes in a way that only simulation and real-life experiences can approximate. A poorly constructed story, on the other hand, leaves learners confused and disengaged.

Most of us recall some challenging clinical situation that can illustrate a point about care. Yet, it may have lost the impact because it was too long ago, we don't remember the details, or we haven't placed the information in a logical sequence. Exhibit 9.1 identifies some ways to initiate adding storytelling to the educator's repertoire of strategies for helping learners learn.

The point of creating a collection of stories and having them categorized is to enable the educator to change the stories so the current class doesn't look like the last one. Using this collection allows the educator to add detail to complex concepts and to substitute for situations that are difficult to reproduce. Thus, not everyone has to deal with end-of-life issues; they can participate

Exhibit 9.1 Creating the Repertoire of Stories

• Record as much detail of a situation as soon after its occurrence as possible.
• Be sure to protect confidential information.
• Be specific about the elements that need details (e.g., a piece of equipment, a specific medication, or a special family member).
• "Overthink" the situation—elements are easier to delete than recall.
• Name the story (see Exhibit 9.2).
• Note if props are needed to make the story effective.
• Date the record to remember if its context is no longer applicable or if it now needs to be a historical story.

Exhibit 9.2 Categories of Stories

1. Historical (the way things were)
2. Values (ethics, patient rights)
3. Interprofessional interactions (conflict resolution, creating effective teams)
4. Workplace issues (violence, staffing)
5. Clinical areas (subdivided to reflect nursing issues, clinical conditions, treatment options, and so forth)
6. Affect of the story (humor, crisis, and so forth)

in a discussion stimulated by a story that allows them to experience the situation from afar. Exhibit 9.2 lists some common categories of stories an educator will use. Depending on typical classroom assignments, other categories can be created to more readily retrieve the stories as they are needed.

================================*FAST FACTS in a NUTSHELL*

- Stories help learners "live" in situations, especially those that are difficult to provide in the clinical or simulation areas.
- Creating a collection allows the educator to keep content fresh and learners engaged.
- Categorizing stories allows an educator to retrieve an appropriate story when needed.

WHAT ARE THE KEY ELEMENTS OF A STORY?

Every good story has a defined beginning ("hook"); middle (the real content); and end (the moral, lesson, main point). Guber (2011, p. 21) describes these elements this way:

- Get your listeners' attention with an unexpected challenge or question.
- Give your listeners an emotional experience by narrating the struggle to overcome the challenge or to find the answer to the opening question.
- Galvanize your listeners' response with an eye-opening resolution that calls *them* to action.

The Beginning

How a story starts sets the tone with which learners listen. Posing a question or making a brief statement about a challenging patient issue quickly grabs their attention and "hooks" them into listening. That opener needs to connect to the purpose of the class session, so it may be important to use words from the class schedule or the daily objective, if one is used. Although every element must be strong, a weak opening may shut down attentiveness, which will be difficult to regain in either of the other elements.

The Middle

The middle is the "meat" of the story. It contains all of the intensity of the situation, it describes the details so learners can place themselves in the same situation vicariously, and it doesn't reveal the ending. This middle part is where the details help learners judge such issues as: Are the lab values normal? Is the nursing assistant performing the task correctly? Does the primary care provider need to be called? Are the vital signs changing as expected? and so forth. These kinds of questions should run through learners' minds when a story is told in sufficient detail to help learners' transport themselves from the classroom to the story's setting. Details of the story such as colors, size, proximity, and specific actions help enliven the engagement with which the learners hear the story.

The End

Finally, the story concludes with the moral of the situation, the resolution of a conflict, the lesson to be learned from specific actions and decisions, and so forth. While our stories may not be eye-opening, they should be so inspiring that learners remember the story as if they had lived it. The ending can lead to a discussion of what other actions might have been taken, an evaluation of the various roles people played in the situation, consideration of what other information would have been helpful to know, or discussion of the interaction of multiple events.

=====*FAST FACTS in a NUTSHELL*

- The "hook" (opening) gets the learner involved from the beginning.
- The middle needs to be detail laden so that the learner feels transported to the situation.
- The end needs to result in some clear message about the purpose of the story so that the learner is clear about the outcome of the story.

WHEN IS THE RIGHT TIME TO TELL STORIES?

Stories can be interspersed throughout a course or a given class session. When they are used depends on their purpose. There are several different types of stories that educators can use to engage learners. Initially educators may be concerned with the amount of time it takes to tell a good story. That makes sense from the experiences most of us have had. However, if the classroom approach is primarily focused on lecture, think about how much more time is consumed in a very passive manner on the part of learners. If learners are not engaged, limited learning is occurring. Benner et al. (2010) call for transforming nursing education so that learners are focused on the patient experience. Telling stories allows learners to hear from the patient, even if the patient isn't available.

The Introductory Story

The introductory story not only allows the educator to provide insight into "who I am" but also sets the tone for how the class will be. In other words, if a usual introduction is made (i.e., "Good morning, I am Dr. Vadis. I am your faculty member for this course . . .") learners receive no message that Dr. Vadis has any added value to the course. Maybe sleeping in later would be better! If the introduction occurs as a story, learners have the opportunity to hear why they should struggle out of bed and spend time in the classroom. Here is an example of a story introduction:

> Have you ever been caught up in a tree? No, I mean really. Of course, I wasn't supposed to be up there and I knew my mother would be really mad. But, for the life of me, I couldn't figure out how to get down! Then it hit me! Spiderman reaches out as far as he can and sticks to the new surface. So, I did. Well, at least the reach part.

That is when I fell and broke my leg. I guessed there was no hiding that from my mother! After the fire department arrived (yes, a neighbor had seen me stranded up in the tree and called the fire department), they rushed me to the hospital, where I met Sammie. Sammie was about nine feet tall and looked like a fullback from Notre Dame. But, Sammie was my nurse. "How could that be?" I remember thinking. Sammie took care of me for the next two days and went with me to the car when my dad came to pick up my mother and me. Sammie whispered in my ear, "You would make a great nurse someday!"

Now the learners know that Dr. Vadis did things he wasn't supposed to do (just like all of us!); that Dr. Vadis had an early experience as a patient, so that may have shaped future plans; and that Dr. Vadis had exposure to a nurse who made a difference—both in the care Dr. Vadis received as a child and in being told about a career expectation.

The Illustrative Story

Throughout a course, educators can use stories to illustrate points. For example, it is much easier to understand some content when examples are given. The closer those examples are to real life, the easier it is to grasp the critical components of the content. Learning about ethics, moral dilemmas, advocacy, and professionalism are examples of content that is a little more nebulous than congestive heart failure or renal failure, and those are complex conditions! Telling a story that illustrates the point the educator wants learners to value helps them see the practical application of what it means to be a nurse. For example, when two Winkler County, Texas, nurses (Yoder-Wise, 2010), Vicki Lynn Galle and Anne Mitchell reported concerns for incompetent practice on the part of a physician, they were investigated, terminated, had charges filed against them, and

one of them went to trial to stand up for nurses' rights to anonymously report unsafe care of patients. Months later, charges
were dropped against Vicki Lynn Galle; and Anne Mitchell was
found not guilty of the charges brought by the county attor-
ney. Hearing Anne and Vicki tell their story puts everybody on
the edge of their seats—even though we may know the ending.
This story, reported in editorials and news columns, makes the
concept of advocacy and leadership very real in terms of what
any of us could do for patients and our community.

The Affective Story

The above example can also be an affective story when the
details of the tribulations are known. Affective stories, however, often don't have as many distracters (such as the legal
aspects). Affective stories help learners gain perspectives on
values, beliefs, attitudes, and appreciation. These stories are
designed to "pull on the heart strings" so that learners gain
perspective on what it means to lose a loved one or a limb or
what it means to face challenging diagnoses. Affective stories
focus much more on the feelings in the situation rather than
the facts. The fact that something happened during a given
week isn't nearly as important as how the person felt and re-
sponded to whatever happened. Using affective domain objectives, especially those at higher levels, helps prepare learners
to face the emotional challenges of being a professional.

The Complexity Story

Educators often focus on one part of a story to make a point.
In real life, though, most stories are complex. There are lots
of facts and comparisons with what is expected to occur.
There are lots of relationship issues—professionals, families,
friends, supporters, and detractors. There are many emotional

aspects; and health issues never occur in isolation from the context of life. A patient preparing for the baptism of a baby while caring for a dying parent, while being out of work and worried about a recalcitrant teenager, can illustrate how a family may live life today. Nothing is simple. So, somewhere in a course, an educator may decide to tell a story of complexity, not to overwhelm learners but to help them gain the perspective that health issues do not happen in isolation. Although our greatest concern may be a diagnosis of cancer, the patient's greatest concern may be for the soul of her grandson. Appreciating that the patient—and the patient's life—are at the core, and highlights that we are merely there to assist with some aspects of life.

═══════════════FAST FACTS in a NUTSHELL

- Stories can be told at any time during the course and serve one of several purposes.
- The introductory story sets the tone for the class in addition to making the educator real.
- The illustrative story is used to make points, especially those that are difficult to understand.
- The affective story engages the attitudes/emotions of the learner to let them "experience" an event or state without being in the actual situation.

HOW DOES ONE CONSTRUCT A GOOD STORY?

First, the message is really important, but that is not the focus of this section. This section focuses on the style or technique for delivering a good story. If an educator has used stories before, maybe focusing on "polishing" the style would make them even more purposeful. If an educator has not used stories before, then focusing on these techniques may create some initial comfort in testing how effective stories are. For both the seasoned and novice storyteller, practice is the most important element. Being able to transition seamlessly from one point to the next keeps learners engaged. Stumbling around (think of the humorist who forgets the punch line of a joke) only makes people anxious, confused, or upset. Practice (and maybe a few notes or props) allows even the lesser experienced storyteller to move readily through a story in a way that makes learners want to know, "What's next?"

Gain the Voice of the Teller

If you are portraying the story as told by a patient, put that person in your mind. Would the patient stand or sit? Would the speaking style be forceful or hesitant? Would the person sound calm and relaxed or anxious and distracted? Is this a young child or an older adult? Your answers determine how you are going to give voice to the story teller.

Use Direct Language

It is very important to actually say the words in the story character's own voice rather than saying something such as, "Mrs. Jones said she was tired of living and needed to lie down." Think how that sounds versus this (in a hushed and hesitant voice): "I . . . I'm so tired of living. I . . . I think I need to lie down." The difference is clear.

Use the "Right" Words

As professionals we might refer to part of the gastrointestinal (GI) track as the colon. Yet few patients, unless they are having a GI procedure, refer to their GI tracks as having parts other than the stomach and bowels. When telling a story, using the words patients use helps learners remember that their task is to meet the patient where the patient is and not to convert the patient into a mini-nurse.

Additionally, if the educator is trying to convey how loud the noise was, it might be appropriate to shout out the next few statements to help make the point. If the educator is trying to "paint a picture," describing sights (colors, sizes, shapes), sounds (type and intensity), aromas (type and intensity), and so forth becomes important. The examples of "it was tart" versus "it was lemony" versus "it was like sucking on a lemon" show how a picture becomes clearer for the listener.

Pacing/Timing

If, for example, the educator wants to convey the anxiety of a situation, increasing the speed of talking helps raise learners' expectations of something intense happening. Alternatively, sometimes pauses are most effective. They can be used to let the last point "hang" for learners so they can reflect on what the point meant. Pausing is also great, especially in combination with shifting the body, to note a transition in time or point. Timing in a story suggests that we place important content throughout the story rather than all in one place. Even if it is logical to group important content, repeating individual elements and drawing them out in more detail can help learners retain what is important.

Tonality

Most people match tonality with their emotions. In other words, few people say "I hate you" with the same tone they would say "I am going to the store." (And when that happens clinically, we have cause for concern!) So, when telling a story, educators may need to shout, whisper, rasp, and so forth. All of this is designed to bring the story alive so the learner is transported into the situation.

Movement

Hand, body, and facial movements are all important. Hands need to match the message and the tonality. Making short, choppy motions when portraying someone who is upset helps learners to get the point: This person is upset. Shifting the body from one side to another or standing "taller" or shrinking all help convey a shift in characters or point, a sense of confidence or hesitancy, and so forth. Even facial movements help tell the story. If the educator is asking a question but looks as if what was just said was a statement of fact, learners get mixed messages about what was said. Sometimes they become so involved in second-guessing themselves ("Did I hear that right?") that they lose the story.

Trivia

Some novelists get carried away with the details and trivia in their story. Sometimes it is so overwhelming that readers put the book down, never to return. That is way too much trivia. However, the idea of trivia, when applied logically, helps learners value the experience the educator is providing. For example, saying "Creeeaaak" (like a squeaky door opening) and then conveying what the nurse said upon entering the patient's room may help astute learners gain the potential to determine that a squeaky door opened many times a day must be a real pain. It is not critical to the story being told. It does, however, enrich the insight into what the patient is experiencing.

==============================*FAST FACTS in a NUTSHELL*

- Practice, practice, practice. Practice helps the educator be more effective in telling a story.
- Movements, tonality, words, and many other aspects comprise the details of telling an effective story.
- "Being the story" as opposed to reporting the story helps learners to be transported into the story.

WHAT SHOULD EDUCATORS EXPECT FROM LEARNERS AFTER THEY HEAR A STORY?

Expectations may vary based on the type of story presented. In general though, learners should have some ideas about what is going on for patients or personnel.

- They should be able to raise questions about what was said by the "characters" in the story.
- They should be able to describe how the class objectives were met through the story.
- They should be able to describe how they felt about the story from the perspective that they were immersed in the details.

Ending a story and then turning to the group with a series of prepared questions can help stimulate the dialogue so that answers are generated from the group with the educator guiding responses. As a result, learners leave with a correct understanding. A beneficial step for the educator to take after the discussion is to summarize both how the story contributed to the objectives of the class session and the broad principles that were applied. Summarizing how the story related to the class objectives and highlighting the principles involved helps learners to value the connections between the principles by which nurses work, the story that demonstrated some objective, and the relevance of the objective to learning.

=====*FAST FACTS in a NUTSHELL*

- Having preplanned questions based on a story can focus the poststory discussion.
- Summarize how the story related to objectives.
- Highlight the principles important to the story and the objectives.

SYNTHESIS

As tough as it is to prepare lectures, telling stories is even more challenging. Being able to have multiple stories to tell to make points clear is a talent to be treasured. Some stories are short and relate to only one or two key-learning elements. Others are complex and pull in various aspects of nursing care. Being able to tell a story so it "comes alive" can be developed through serious practice in telling the story and assuming the voice of the patient. The value of stories is that they can transport learners to a situation they might not logically encounter and yet is important for them professionally. Stories engage learners—and for that matter, the educator—and contribute to our deeper understanding of what is known as the patient experience.

PART

IV

Dialogue Toward Improvement

10

Creating Standard Communication

The journey of discovery should not include reading the educator's mind. Clear communications allows the learner to get on with the business of learning, while allowing the details to remain in the background. Sometimes that requires having standard messages a group of educators decide is useful for all learners. Sharing information includes sharing expectations both of what we expect of the learner AND what the learner can expect from us.

Fran Vlasses, PhD, NEA-BC, ANEF, FAAN

INTRODUCTION

Unlike scripting, a practice used in many health care organizations, standard communication refers to common responses educators need to use to be consistent from one learner to another and from one educator to another. We all know this game, probably because we played it as children. If I don't like answer one, I will go ask the other parent. Sometimes learners are not doing this as a game but rather to hear the response in a way that makes sense

to them. If they don't hear the same essence, they become
confused and anxious, and in some cases, manipulative.
Creating standard communication is designed to over-
come the potential downsides of explanations.

In this chapter, you will learn:

1. The rationale for standard communication
2. Who needs to be involved in the development and use of standard communication
3. Some common and needed standard communications
4. How to employ standard communication

WHAT IS THE RATIONALE FOR USING STANDARD COMMUNICATION?

In most nursing programs, an educator does not function in isolation. Singular course assignments are rare, so that means a team of educators work together to implement a given course. Once there is more than one person in a given course or class, some coordination of communication needs to occur. If educators haven't worked out in advance what words such as *timely, prompt, accurate, appropriate, neat,* and so forth mean, learners can quickly discern the differences of opinions about what those terms mean and, in some cases, use the differences to their advantage and to the disadvantage of the educator. The up-front intensity of sorting through such elements (or the avoidance of such terms in the first place) creates less hassle as the course or class progresses, and it prevents diversion of the conversation from what is really important in nursing to a sidebar conversation about "how prompt does prompt need to be?" in order to meet the expectation of promptness.

What Comprises "Standard Communication"?

This decision rests with educators. A common way to determine what needs to be standardized is to determine what elements precipitate the greatest number of questions from learners. Another is to think about when a learner argued about the outcome of an assignment. What was said that could lead the educator to determine that some term needed to be standardized? Common examples were cited in the beginning of this section. These are terms that commonly require professional judgment; however, they may translate to novice learners as capricious rather than as "taking into account a number of variables." (And that is an example of standard communication!) Standard communication does not mean all educators must say the same exact words and repeat those words over and over. Rather, standard communication means that the team of educators has a mutual agreement about what are potentially confusing words so that the bottom-line message means the same. The example below shows how two different educators hold the same conversation using different words and concluding with the same bottom-line message.

Learner: I can't get to the clinical area until 8:15 a.m. [clinical starts at 8 a.m.].

Educator: The syllabus [note the reference to an official document] states that promptness is expected. That means 8:15 would be unacceptable.

Learner: Well, maybe I could get there by about 8:10.

Educator: I appreciate your thinking through what is possible and the result I hear still doesn't meet the expectation.

Learner: Well, how late can I be and still be prompt?

Educator: "Late" is not part of the expectation of promptness. I imagine that being late would actually mean arriving at 8 because the expectation is you are ready to begin your work at 8.

(Learner goes to another educator.)

Learner: I can't get to the clinical area until 8:15 a.m. [clinical starts at 8 a.m.].

Educator 2: You must have a lot going on for yourself right now. [Learner interrupts.]

Learner: You have no idea. My mother isn't able to take care of my kids and my babysitter comes from across town and my husband doesn't get home until about a quarter to 8 and . . . [Educator signals "stop"].

Educator 2: I understand how tough life can be at certain points. The clinical starts at 8 a.m. and promptness means you need to be there and ready to go. Would you like for me to think through options for promptness with you?

Clearly the two educators are taking two different approaches, but the bottom line message is this: be there by 8 a.m. and ready to work. When educators agree, the learners become clear.

═══════════════*FAST FACTS in a NUTSHELL*

- Standard communication decreases the confusion when multiple educators work with multiple learners.
- Making the same general statements reinforces that those messages are the official ones.
- Standard communication prevents difficult situations when a learner hears different messages from different educators.

WHO NEEDS TO BE INVOLVED IN CREATING STANDARD COMMUNICATIONS?

Probably the ideal would be for an entire group of educators to create standard communications. Realistically, it may be the individual or a group of educators in a given course.

If the group changes, new members of the group need to know about the standard communication and at a minimum, accept its use for the current learning experience. Terms can be changed as can the standard messages. Changes actually may be a good thing. Changes don't necessarily suggest a waffling on what something means. Changes may reflect a better appreciation of the numerous interpretations that were made with the use of the previously agreed-to standard communication. This information suggests that the group (all or some) would evaluate the perceived outcomes of the standard communication so that changes could be made if necessary.

So, if the whole program doesn't have standard communication, how does one educator (or a group) implement this strategy without alienating others or conveying to learners that someone else was wrong not to have such? Again, standard communication can help. Prefacing responses with phrases such as "the syllabus states" or "in this course, this means" makes clear that the absence of a bigger perspective does not negate what happens in a particular course. Pointing out to learners that differences exist between courses might even be a good thing! In the real world of nursing, not all policies in all organizations have the same meaning. This variance allows learners to experience adaptability.

Even when one educator has "my course" and others are introduced, some mutual understanding of what the standard communication needs to be must occur. A self-assured educator asks the newcomers for their input into those communications. If that doesn't occur, the newcomers should convey they want to know what those communications are so that they can contribute to the standard of the course. Realistically, some assignments to courses occur at the last minute and the educator arriving into the course basically needs a "cheat sheet" of what it means to be in that course. If the current individual educator or team doesn't have this information, the newcomer can indicate how valuable this will be—and thus immediately help the team, even if it doesn't feel like help initially—and state what those terms mean personally to the newcomer so that others can provide feedback if the understanding isn't correct.

======*FAST FACTS in a NUTSHELL*

- The ideal situation is to have all educators who work together on similar work provide input and agree about what the standard communication is.
- Sometimes timing prevents input, so the focus is on making certain all the educators understand what the standard communication is and what its value is to a specific course.

WHAT ARE SOME COMMON AND NEEDED COMMUNICATIONS?

Exhibit 10.1 presents some common terms that can trap educators and thus are worthy of a mutual understanding. That understanding has no judgment about right or wrong; it is merely a consensus of the educators about what the term will mean. Sometimes these terms are dealt with in a course evaluation rubric; other times, they are not. The nursing program may have common definitions; however, the lack of such should not prevent an educator or group from creating what the educator or group needs. The clearer a group—or even an individual—can be, the lesser the chance for multiple interpretations and the subsequent consequences. The more evident this standard language is to learners, the more useful it is for educators to abide by those messages. Even putting the standard communication in a syllabus may be useful.

Another example of standard communication is the kind that learners need to know so well that when they hear the standard message, they know what is expected of them. For example, the strategy known as "think/pair/square/share" (Bain, 2004) could be defined in the syllabus. The faculty

Exhibit 10.1   Common Terms That Need Standard Communication

Timely

Prompt

Accurate

Appropriate

Neat

Nursing Standards

Complete

Due Date

Exhibit 10.2   Think/Pair/Square/Share Strategy

Think: Take a few minutes to think about what you were asked to consider.

Pair: At the designated time, turn to a colleague sitting nearby and discuss your two perspectives.

Square: At the designated time, each pair pairs with another pair so that there are four people in discussion.

Share: At the designated time, each square is eligible to offer comments on the thinking and discussion that occurred on the topic.

Source: Adapted from Bain (2004).

member could then simply say something such as: "In order to consider the implications of this information, let's think/pair/square/share." The syllabus might include the information regarding this strategy, as shown in Exhibit 10.2.

====================================*FAST FACTS in a NUTSHELL*

- Even if common standard communication is not used by the program, individual educators or groups can create their own.

HOW IS STANDARD COMMUNICATION EMPLOYED?

Basically, standard communication sets the edges or the boundaries on a given term or topic. Because learners learn from multiple perspectives, using both printed words (such as the syllabus) and oral words (such as an introductory agreement or standards-setting activity) helps learners gain the perspective of what the expectations mean for them. The idea that educators would meet in advance of a course adds strain to busy schedules, but it produces greater synergy among the educators as they work together over a period of time.

Some educators will feel more comfortable sticking only to the standard communication and using the "broken-record technique" of repeating the same words over and over again. For example, as a learner argues about a point, the educator simply says: "I understand and the expectation for neatness applies to all settings." When the learner continues to argue his or her point, the educator says the exact same words again. Other educators will feel more comfortable varying the message while incorporating the standard communication. For example, as the same learner argues a point, the educator says: "That is a good point, and yet the expectation for neatness applies across the board to all settings in which you are involved." When the learner continues to argue the point, the educator says: "I can hear you are really passionate about this and some places do use different expectations for neatness. Ours does not. The expectation for neatness is the same in any setting we use." Note that even though the words aren't always the same, the message is!

Whenever one educator says to another, "Wait till you hear this one," it is a signal that alerts both to the potential need for standard communication. Generally speaking, we all know the usual issues requiring absolute consistency among a group of educators (refer to Exhibit 10.1 again to review those issues). Walking the fine line between being helpful to the learner who truly needs an exception made, and being manipulated by the learner who went to a party last night rather than completing an assignment, is a challenge. Standard communication helps deal with both situations because there is a common reference point. Even if an educator is working in a setting where things such as deadlines aren't important, the competencies/standards are. Again, standard communication helps all educators convey the same message to all learners.

═══════════════════════════════════════FAST FACTS in a NUTSHELL

- Variance in style of communication may make the message seem more personalized.
- Agreeing to and implementing the standard communication helps educators work with learners who attempt to vary the expectations and standards.

SYNTHESIS

If educators don't have the need for defined expectations, creating standard communication may not be beneficial. For those, however, who work with learners who want certain conditions, expectations, or standards varied based on their specific needs, standard communication can be highly valuable. The more up-front about the specifics of the expectation, the less resistance might occur.

II

Seeking Input

*Around the fourth week of the semester I have
learners "Take the Course Temperature." I ask what is
going well and what might need to be changed. Based
on the "hot" and "not so hot" comments, I have made
some immediate changes in courses. End of semester
comments also have led to course improvement.
Without question, learner comments have made me
a much better educator. Listen to your learners if you
want to improve your teaching!*

Betsy Frank, PhD, RN, ANEF

INTRODUCTION

Many educators value imparting knowledge to others.
That is a good thing based on the role they have chosen.
Equally important, however, is gaining input from the
learners. Gaining input and imparting knowledge are
complementary yet different strategies. Gaining input
often requires that educators draw on numerous resources to be prepared for a class session. In other words,
it is not possible to rely on allocating some number of
minutes per page of notes or per PowerPoint slide. Now
the educator needs to be ready to go where the learners'

> *input steers. When one seeks ongoing input, it is like a work in progress. In short, learning evolves. Educators are always guided by the anticipated outcomes; how they get there, however, may be as varied as a mosaic or tapestry. Being highly competent is an asset, but it is not a necessity. Being comfortable, however, with responses that acknowledge voids in content is a critical skill.*

In this chapter, you will learn:

1. The reasons for seeking input
2. The strategies and timing for seeking input
3. The value of seeking input

REASONS FOR SEEKING INPUT

When education consisted of "the sage on the stage," we could easily blame learners for not grasping critical information. After all, "I told them what they needed to know. They must not have listened." In a blame-free culture, however, the point is to focus on what we can do in the best possible way. Educators need to facilitate learning and learners need to engage in that learning and let educators know when something is unclear or when questions remain. That two-way exchange is critical for productive learning. As Benner et al. suggested, "nursing learners need to learn for a practice, and every class should contribute to their clinical imagination" (2010, p. 79). Thus, the obligation of educators is to create discussions that focus on complex, challenging, and critical clinical scenarios that, in essence, transport learners to the clinical area so that they can envision what the patient looks like, how he or she would respond, what the pathology has caused as physical and physiological changes, and what the person's mental health, social health, and family health status is like. As a result, learners are freed to be imaginative in their solutions to the challenges they will face in the real practice of nursing.

If we are not seeking input from learners, we have no way of knowing what their learning is like, if they see the crucial elements in a situation, if they can adapt their attention when some nuance redirects their thinking, or if their clinical reasoning skills are faulty. If we are not seeking input from learners throughout the learning process, we also might feel defensive when something doesn't work. In part this is because we didn't know where the learners were in relation to what the expectations were. By having learners involved in ongoing input, they not only influence the progress of a learning experience but also gain assessment skills that can be transferred to future situations—for example, self-evaluations.

The most common way we assess learning is through testing. Yet, most tests are construed as multiple choice options. As challenging as it is to produce a high-quality test, those examinations force a decision among selected options. While that strategy mimics the licensure and certification examinations, it does not mimic the clinical setting where endless options are available and where, without sufficient grounding, any element can be viewed as critical.

The richer the educator can make the classroom experience in terms of creating the clinical experiences, the greater the work commitment and the greater the positive outcomes for learning. Seeking input is a strategy to help learners build their assessment skills, something that is a critical behavior throughout nursing.

========================*FAST FACTS in a NUTSHELL*

- Seeking input throughout a course helps educators adjust what they do to meet learners' needs.
- The goal of effective classroom teaching is to enhance learners' clinical reasoning skills.

STRATEGIES AND TIMING OF SEEKING INPUT

For input to be valuable to the present learners, input cannot consist solely of end-of-course evaluation. That evaluation is highly useful for considerations about what to do for the future. However, it is a terminal process. It doesn't benefit the current set of learners. It doesn't promote active adjustments to making content clearer, hearing different views of a topic, or devising additional or optional approaches to learning complex content. Rather, an ongoing evaluation can be garnered by seeking input from learners on some regular schedule. That schedule might be at each class session, at a calendar interval, or some other schemata. As early as 1967, the idea of using both summative (end of course) *and* formative (during the course) evaluation was posed (Scriven, 1967). Yet, except for testing, some educators still do not use a planned approach to formative input to determine the extent to which learners are grasping the complexities of the content. Some of these questions might relate to the classroom climate. For example, the educator might ask if everyone can see something on a screen, whiteboard, or flipchart or the patient at the front of the room. Yet, the real questions relate to the learning process. As Benner et al. (2010) made clear, learners need to be actively engaged by responding to questions and working through clinical case studies in order to reach the higher level of cognitive and affective objectives the profession of nursing demands of its practitioners.

When an educator asks a question, for example, the learner's response can provide data about the learner's perception of the situation. If the educator uses deliberative group involvement, such as a case study, listening to the emphasis on critical elements and omission of extraneous details is important. What both of these approaches do is help the educator know the effectiveness of the learning thus far. Note that what the educator is focusing on is the learning rather than on whether the learning is derived from a film, a lecture, a text, an online source, or the clinical setting. In other words, the source, unless it is questionable, is not the important element. Learning is the important element.

Seeking Input at the Beginning of a Class Session

Creating the classroom situation so that learners must provide input enhances learner engagement and educator modifications or reinforcements. The following scenario illustrates how to establish the situation at the beginning of a class session for providing feedback.

> *Educator:* Thank you all for turning in your worksheets for today. You may recall that we are going to be focusing on a case study today involving an 89-year-old man with COPD. Again, this was case study number 3 from your syllabus. So, let's all decide what we would want to do before we called this patient into the clinic area. Feel free to volunteer.
>
> *Learner A:* Well, because the basic problem is breathing, I would want to be sure that we had a fairly odor-free room available for him. And, I'd want to check the record to see if he had stopped smoking, or if he had been a smoker. I also would want to know what his drugs were and what kind of pulmonary rehab he might be engaged in. Some of that was included in the case study.
>
> *Learner B:* I think the big thing is to find out how he thinks he is doing with his chronic health problem. He is coming in for a routine visit, not for some specific problem. I want to know what his activity level is like, if he is enjoying life, if he is cognitively connected. I know that one of the co-morbidities is depression. I want to be sure that isn't present for him because there was nothing cited about that in the case study.
>
> *Learner C:* If I remember correctly, the pathology of COPD interferes with energy effectiveness in the body. I would be very interested in his current weight and that was not part of the case study in the syllabus. I'd also want to know if he

could easily walk to the clinic area or if we needed to provide assistance.

Educator: Good point, let me pull up some weight data so that you can see if any changes exist and if so, what the trend is.

Learner D: While you are doing that, I wanted to say I would check to see if his sputum had blood in it.

Learner A: I don't think that is associated with COPD. We want to check for color but it is more to see if there is an infection. Blood is associated with some other condition.

Learner B: One of those is TB.

Educator: Thanks for carrying on the discussion while I pulled up the weight data. First, you are right that what we want to check for in the sputum is a change in color and that change is not associated with blood. We probably wouldn't do a sputum test unless the patient conveyed something to us that made us think there was a change. We could ask, as an example, if he looks at anything he coughs up. This would help us know if he is trying to expectorate what he produces and what he is seeing when he does. Let's look at the weight data now. What point made us want to know this?

That scenario illustrates how learners can interact among themselves with little involvement from the educator and still get to the right information. In fact, this example shows how the group itself corrects information. Before this exchange can happen, however, the educator needs to set the expectation for such discussion. In the example above, what the educator has learned thus far is that as a group, learners are seeing the case study from a fairly holistic perspective. The educator also now knows that Learner D is confused or unable to accurately recall important information about the condition of COPD. That feedback could allow the educator to use a learning prescription to help Learner D gain a more in-depth understanding of what the pathophysiology of COPD is, so that the learner's nursing actions are based on scientific knowledge.

Seeking Input During a Class Session

During the class session, educators need to stimulate evaluation of the ideas that learners present or that were presented to them. Sometimes that can be accomplished by merely asking a question at various points to cause learners to pause and evaluate what just transpired. Another strategy, however, is a little more complex and engages all in the evaluation activity. This is illustrated in the following scenario:

> *Educator:* We have been spending some time now planning out the various elements of care for this community. Let's stop and evaluate where what we have said is taking us. If you would return to your usual subgroup [this assumes this strategy has been used before and that there was a formal declaration of the subgroups], let's look at our anticipated outcomes. I am allotting 5 minutes for the subgroups to create evaluative statements that we will share with the whole group to decide if we are being effective in our approach.

Another approach an educator might use during a class session is to ask the learners to make a few statements about their learning thus far. This could be accomplished by having learners send the educator an e-mail related to what they are experiencing or by having them use a standard form to indicate their perceptions of their learning. What is important is to help learners gain insight into assessing their own learning and decisions so that the process might transfer to clinical settings. In other words, the educator is helping the learner develop useful skills even though that is not the "content" of the class session. If this activity is done in writing, it allows the educator to provide specific and focused feedback to aid the learner in being more precise either about the content or the process or both. Asking, "And how can we make it better?" might elicit suggestions to strengthen the strategy. Asking learners to evaluate their own learning creates an expectation that this is an ongoing professional behavior to be carried on throughout their professional lives.

Seeking Input at the End of the Class Session

Equally important is how to gain input at the end of any class session. One technique, known as the "one-minute paper," was described in the Harvard Assessment Seminars (Light, 1986). See Chapter 8, p. 116 for more details. This technique consists of learners answering two questions. The educator asks learners to take a sheet of paper (note that this might require some advanced planning based on the fact that some of today's learners operate almost exclusively in an electronic environment). The educator can state the questions, or write them on a whiteboard or show a slide with the questions. Learners are to answer these two questions anonymously.

The first question is designed to determine the learners' grasp of the content of the day. The question can be worded as, "What was the big point of class today?" or a variation thereof.

The second question is designed to learn more about the concerns learners have related to what they think they missed or didn't comprehend. This question can be worded as, "What question remains?" or a variation thereof.

Exhibit 11.1 is a helpful reminder to the educator to conclude the sessions with the big point and the big question. Just by keeping a card with those two symbols can remind educators to gain this input at the close of each interaction.

Essentially, in one minute, each learner can write brief responses to those two questions, turn the sheet of paper in on exiting, or leave the sheet at the seat. The educator collects the sheets and then creates answers for the questions

Exhibit 11.1   Big Point/Big Question

that remain or comments for the big point. This information can be shared online prior to the next class session or prepared as a handout to be distributed at the next class session. Sharing the information online is especially useful if there is a time delay between class sessions. That way, learners receive clarification and have the knowledge they need to build on for their next endeavor.

Sharing the big points can be helpful to each learner from at least a couple of perspectives. The first is that learners now have a repertoire of what is important that is broader than their individual responses. The second is that learners can gain an appreciation that there are many ways to see a situation and what is important in it.

Sharing the responses to questions is easy when the questions are factual in nature. What is the normal A1C value? That is an example of an easily addressed response. Sometimes the questions are more complex. For example, a learner might respond to a session about ethics with this question: "How do you make our local hospital change when it is clear they don't support nursing's Code of Ethics?" This is not a simple change–type response. The educator has to know if the learner's perception of the local hospital is accurate. Does the hospital have a code of ethics that incorporates various professional codes? Is the nursing code's information imbedded in the hospital's various policies? Or, is it in fact ignored? Is there lack of support or merely an oversight? What is the nature of change needed based on the assessment of the local hospital? It is not possible to address these numerous questions that might emerge for any given learner response. Thus, this example might cause the educator to suggest that a clinical conference be devoted to the topic or that the next clinical scenario be adjusted so that there is more of a discussion about ethics and their importance in the clinical area. Similarly, if there were numerous questions about people who have diabetes, the wise educator might create a learning module or direct learners to a specific resource for more information.

The above is the "short view" of the situation, that is, how to deal with the immediacy of the big point and big question. An adjustment can be made immediately when it is clear there is something missing for several learners that cannot readily be answered by a short sentence or paragraph. The wise educator tracks this type of input when learning experiences are repeated to determine if consistent input suggests a specific action is needed. Additionally, the educator can initiate the next class session by referring to the prior one, as illustrated in this next scenario.

> *Educator:* Thank you again for turning in your worksheets. I posted my responses to your input about the big point and big question on the website and directed you to some additional resources. First, I want to commend you all for grasping how complex the condition known as diabetes is. It was clear that from all of the responses, you saw the priorities of concern and the holistic impact this chronic condition has on people and their families. Before we move forward in the syllabus, I want us to clarify what I thought was some confusion about the nursing actions we needed to be prepared to take. So let's pull up our prior case study and review again what the critical cues were for us to take action. Let's work in small groups . . .

In that scenario, the educator returned to clarify misperceptions related to the prior session's discussion. Know that when we do this, we may feel anxious. Less time is now available for the content that was to be covered in the current session. The question educators need to decide is which is better: to move ahead with additional new content, or to return to content that caused confusion for several learners so that misinformation is diminished or eliminated? It is not possible to always return in depth to a prior discussion, but information that is incorrect needs to be called out so that no one leaves the room thinking that the inaccurate information was okay.

Seeking Input at the End of a New Activity/Strategy

Innovative educators introduce new ways of learning on a fairly regular basis. We get instant feedback (the frowns and smiles) regarding how the activity or strategy was received. If our goal as educators is to always do our best, it isn't sufficient to introduce and then use the new strategy. Rather, we must also ask basic questions such as, "How did you think this helped you learn about people who live with osteomylitis?" By seeking information about the process itself, the educator learns potential ways to improve on the technique in later sessions of the course or in subsequent courses. Gaining insight into how the learners see the activity is important because if it is not strengthening their knowledge and ability to apply that knowledge, it was just "nice to know"—and most curricula have little or no room for that in the core efforts of learning.

═══════════════════════*FAST FACTS in a NUTSHELL*

- Educators can employ specific strategies at various points in a class session to stimulate input from the learners.
- Providing validation of correct information and correction of incorrect information is important when no opportunity is present for further discussion and when the information is fairly straightforward.
- Correcting complex information that is misunderstood is a justification to alter the next class session if sufficient numbers of learners had misperceptions of content.

VALUE OF SEEKING INPUT

We all know that learners learn in different ways, and there are some clear-cut facts we must know. Further, we know that the thinking required for nurses is a complex process involving multiple sciences to emerge as the dynamic nurse–patient interaction. How then can we know what is going on for learners unless we seek their input on an ongoing basis so that we can adjust the rapidity and complexity of the learning situation? The emphasis on "so much to cover" is an important factor. However if we simply "cover" content without understanding the learner experience, we can be finished with a course and not have produced much high-level learning.

- Relying on clinical alone usually is insufficient, if the ratios of educators to learners aren't narrowly defined.
- Relying on simulation alone is insufficient, if the experience doesn't incorporate some intense time with high-fidelity learning.
- Relying on texts or online programming alone is insufficient, if there isn't an opportunity to explore, validate, and correct information.
- Relying on the "traditional" classroom approach is insufficient, if there isn't the opportunity to engage learners in providing input so that their knowledge can be validated or corrected.

Learners may convey messages that make it clear that they don't like a specific activity. The job of the educator is to address that issue and not necessarily to cave in to pressures from the learners. Thus, the educator might say something such as, "We will continue using groups that I construct. Let me tell you why. In the real world, few teams get to create themselves. Rather, they are created by someone and then have to learn how to work together as a team to accomplish the group's goals." An explanation such as that may not dissuade some learners from continuing to give voice to concerns about the nature of the teams, but now the educator has a context in which to address their concerns. The point is the educator conveyed the idea of hearing the concern while simultaneously adhering to the necessary plan.

The purpose of seeking input, as stated earlier, is to engage the learner so that formative evaluations about the progress of the course can be made. That progress is expected to enhance learners' clinical reasoning skills so that they are better able to interact effectively in patient care situations than if they did not have such support.

FAST FACTS in a NUTSHELL

- Seeking input throughout a course allows educators to adjust the learning experiences to be more effective in helping learners to develop solid clinical reasoning skills.

SYNTHESIS

Rather than filling the class time with content, the goal for educators is to create space for learning. Included in that goal is the idea of educators seeking input from learners in a planned way. While this approach engages the learners in active processes, the point here is that educators are gaining insight into what learners are learning and what corrections to the planned learning experiences need to be made. The strategies to elicit input from learners need to be employed throughout the course and be so commonplace that learners can easily transition into the input activities. This type of formative evaluation allows educators to make sound decisions related to altering or continuing their plans for learning. Educators have a grasp of what learners know, how they can use it when presented with clinical replica, and what needs to be refocused. Seeking input strengthens the learning experience and the educator's ability to be an effective facilitator for learning.

12

Providing Feedback

The educator's feedback to learners is an important factor in their learning. Feedback is the specific information that the educator provides to learners to guide their learning; with this information, learners know what they still need to learn to be successful. Feedback should be continuous and instructional, woven in the teaching process.

Marilyn H. Oermann, PhD, RN, FAAN, ANEF

INTRODUCTION

Equally important to seeking input from learners is providing them with feedback. Feedback accomplishes several things: It creates connections for the learner, it redirects any erroneous thoughts, it reinforces solid clinical reasoning, and it serves as a way for the educator to make observations about the learner and the learner's progress. Feedback can be achieved in many ways. In order to assure that feedback occurs, it is important to incorporate it into the basic planning for any learning activity. Feedback needs to be nonjudgmental if it is to produce the most positive results for future

163

activities. This is an important consideration because many people view feedback negatively. When feedback focuses on the opportunity to improve, no matter where learners are on a performance scale, they now have more information about improvement.

In this chapter, you will learn:

1. What purpose feedback serves
2. How feedback improves learning
3. What strategies are effective in providing feedback
4. How debriefing works

THE PURPOSE OF FEEDBACK

Providing feedback to learners as a group and as individuals is a critical part of the educator's role. Most learners take some action because they think that is the best action to take. They are trying to do the right thing. If what is being done isn't correct or if it is okay but could be better, learners are unlikely to change without some form of feedback. And, if they are doing something correctly, unless educators ask the rationale behind the action, the decision to do one thing versus another may have been happenstance. So, these learners too need feedback to continue the correct behavior.

Some learners gain insight of the need to change by reading something that redirects their behavior. Most learners, however, need the added assistance of feedback to encourage them toward new behaviors.

- Providing feedback can set learners on the track of best practices.
- If the learner is already "there," feedback can reinforce the importance of the behaviors.

- If the learner doesn't have a clue where to begin, feed-back can help the learner approach the content needed.

The following examples illustrate feedback that might be helpful in each of those cases:

> **Poor Practice.** *The learner poses a response that is not correct in the given situation.*
>
> *Learner:* I would give the patient his insulin right away.
>
> *Educator:* What might you want to do before you administered any insulin?
>
> **Correct Practice.** *The learner poses a response that is the best practice in a given situation.*
>
> *Learner:* I think we need to advocate for carbonated beverages to be removed from the vending machines.
>
> *Educator:* What source of literature suggests this is a good action to take?
>
> **Uninformed.** *The learner doesn't know what a possible action might be.*
>
> *Educator:* Let's assume that we needed to administer some oxygen for this patient. What do you know about when and why we do that?

========================*FAST FACTS in a NUTSHELL*

- People usually try to do the right thing.
- Without feedback, people continue to do what they have done before.

HOW FEEDBACK IMPROVES LEARNING

The goal of providing feedback is to help reinforce positive behaviors and to redirect or modify negative ones. Feedback, in essence, answers questions such as:

- How am I doing?
- What could I do better or differently?
- What is the rationale for thinking as I did?

Feedback can provoke the imagination. In other words, the educator can pose the "what ifs" for a situation that result in a more complex clinical issue. For learners who are close to completing a program, this is especially useful (although the technique can be used throughout). Now instead of thinking, for example, of a patient with a dual diagnosis, learners are provoked to consider what will happen if the family is not supportive of the patient, or if the patient lives miles from healthcare access, or if an injury occurs for the patient's primary care giver. This kind of provocation builds on an initial conversation of feedback related to the original case discussion.

Additionally, once learners become engaged in receiving feedback, they may become more comfortable in providing it. Then the educator can create deliberate opportunities where learners can give and receive feedback. The educator, for example, might pose three case studies for evaluation and indicate that everyone has the opportunity to comment on one unless he or she is motivated to do more and receive and give more feedback. This allows learners who want to test their reasoning skills to have more practice without setting a goal that is frustrating for those who don't have that same desire.

Overcoming Obstacles in Providing Feedback

In some situations, learners are too anxious to hear what the educator says. In others, they may be too blasé. These are some extremes of what interferes with learners receiving the messages provided to them. Effective feedback is designed to help learners engage with the messages rather than "get the answer and go" or remain in a state of nonreceptivity.

In the two extremes (anxious and blasé) presented above, one of the most effective strategies is to acknowledge what is sensed.

- For example, the educator might start by saying something such as: "I can almost feel the tension in the room. I think many of you are anxious. Would someone correct my perception if I am wrong?" If that question is followed by silence, the educator can first acknowledge that their silence means the perception was right and then further explore the nature of the anxiety and focus on what learners can do to decrease their anxiety. Even in large groups, the educator might want to say: "Write this down" and then proceed to define a mnemonic to help learners remember some important information that they need to have to solve a clinical issue.
- Another example might be to have learners create a diagram or picture representing some critical information to help them recall the important information that they need to have to solve a clinical issue. An educator might also encourage mind maps.

In the situation where the learners were blasé, the educator's strategy is to create a compelling case around which the learners can rally. The experienced educator likely has more than one case study as an example, and can switch from one that might be more simplistic to one that is more complex so that different groups have to work on different aspects. Storytelling is also effective for many learners in this situation because suddenly the discussion is about someone specific, not someone in the abstract.

FAST FACTS in a NUTSHELL

- Feedback shapes behavior.
- The educator needs to deal with the emotional climate in a group before moving to key content.

EFFECTIVE FEEDBACK STRATEGIES

Some examples have already been given here and throughout the book. If learners are anxious, first reduce their anxiety. If they are blasé, first get them engaged. If they are open to learning, ask them questions. The goal of education is to help learners learn, not to provide content. Let us say that again: **the goal of education is to help learners learn, not to provide content**. That may sound a little trite; however, many educators are focused on content, what to put in the Power-Point presentation, what the test questions must be, and so forth—rather than on what does the educator need to do to help learners figure out resources, correct answers, and better thinking strategies to get to the content. The activity below is designed to help educators recall or rethink what strategies they might use to provide effective feedback.

Activities

Look at the table of contents. Ask if there is something in each of the chapters that helps with providing feedback. Just place a checkmark beside each chapter number for now. Now go back and make a note of the idea you gained from the chapter that could allow you to give feedback.

Examples

Agreements: (Chapter 4)

A learner violates the agreement about not texting on the phone during the class session.

The educator responds by handing a note that says "AGREEMENT" on it. This was the agreed-to manner of an early warning regarding using cell phones in class.

A learner continues to violate the agreement about not texting after receiving the written note.

The educator responds by handing a note that says "Please leave. Return when you are ready to be part of the group."

The learner returns to the classroom and once again is observed using the phone to text.

This time the educator stops the class and approaches the learner and says "You remember that our agreement was that no cell phones would be used in the classroom. Is there an emergency that prevents your living up to the agreement? If not, this is a violation of the trust of the group. How will you regain it?" (Remember that the goal here is to reinforce accountability, a professional value, and not to embarrass, although this situation may be an embarrassment.)

Questions: (Chapter 8)

A learner provides a response that is accurate and also not the best practice.

The educator responds by asking: "What could be a newer approach to providing that care?"

Coaching: (Chapter 7)

A learner is orally reflecting on the care he provided in the clinical assignment the day before. He is providing details about the intensity of the various things he did.

The educator responds by asking: "I would feel really tense in that situation. How did you feel?"

The learner responds, and the educator then asks: "What other situations might be like that?"

Standard Communication: (Chapter 10)

Learners want to form their own groups.

The educator responds by saying: "No, that isn't how it happens in the real world. In the real world, you have to figure out how to make things work with the group you are in, not the group you desire to be in."

Learners want an extension at the end of the course for a project that is due.

The educator responds by saying: "The syllabus identifies that late projects are accepted and that 5 points are deducted for each day the project is late. You certainly have the choice of submitting the project after the deadline, and the consequences can be found on page 5 of the syllabus."

FAST FACTS in a NUTSHELL

- The goal of education is to help learners learn, not to provide content.
- Consider how to use the various strategies in this book as ways to provide feedback.

USING DEBRIEFING

Feedback provides the opportunity to debrief a situation. It is reflective practice in action. For example, an educator may have role-played a situation with one of the learners. After it is concluded and the learner is acknowledged for being willing to participate, the educator can use the strategy of debriefing to help all learners learn from the example provided. The educator might begin by having the risk-taking learner share with the group what assuming that role felt like. The affective domain expectations and performance can be discussed. After addressing the affective domain, the educator might turn to the cognitive domain and ask the group if there were better responses or if they knew sources that could document the actions taken. The educator could also ask what the most effective action was in the role-play situation and what the least effective action was. After various aspects are discussed, the educator could then ask what a concluding comment about the role-play interaction might be.

═══════════════════════════════*FAST FACTS in a NUTSHELL*

- Debriefing is reflection in action.
- Debriefing can effectively incorporate the affective domain.

SYNTHESIS

Feedback is a critical element in the learning process. Whether it is where to place a napkin at a meal, when to initiate a given therapy with a patient, or when to call a physician in the middle of the night, without feedback we continue to do what we did before. Providing negative feedback is either off-putting (as in why a mother said how to place a napkin in a specific way), or unsafe (as in if the physician derides a nurse for disturbing the physician's sleep). Positive feedback reinforces positive behaviors, and feedback said in a positive manner helps us better approximate the most positive behaviors.

PART

V

Synthesis

13

Integrating the Whole

I've had the privilege of being a nurse educator for over 25 years. As an educator, I've had the honor of facilitating, mentoring, and teaching thousands of individuals as they progressed in their career as a nurse. Reflecting on the past I am fortunate to have discovered my passion for teaching early in my career. Being a nurse educator allowed me to impact health care delivery both directly through my personal involvement and indirectly through each of my learners. Looking back, the one constant has been change and being an excellent educator correlated directly with my ability to embrace change. Looking forward . . . envisioning our future we need to ask . . . "Where will nursing be in 25 years?" or better stated "What is the role nursing envisions for itself in the future?" "What transformation is required in nursing education to prepare our graduates for this future?" and "How can I lead this transformation?" I think being integrative, pulling on all of my strengths, helps me be my best in every encounter and I count on that for the future.

Sharon Decker, PhD, RN, ANEF, FAAN

INTRODUCTION

Although learners often voice dissatisfaction with having to think for themselves, most learners clearly understand the rationale for why they must be actively engaged. Learners may be concerned with providing the right responses to questions or coming prepared to participate. They could be concerned about the clarity of expectations for the learning activities and outcomes. One of the critical elements that an educator must execute well is creating the whole learning experience so that the strengths of learners are used to help them be better at providing care to patients. Decreasing learner anxiety, making clear what will happen next, providing opportunities for input into the ongoing progress of a course, and providing support to explore how to reach conclusions about nursing actions in various roles are examples of what the educator must attend to.

The first 12 chapters provided content about various strategies that help the educator facilitate learning by the learners. Each chapter's content is valuable in itself, yet integrating each element with the others can seem overwhelming for those educators who were not prepared to teach in this manner. An analogy might be helpful.

> Many of us know about the various steps in playing golf. Stance is important, how to hold the club is important, where to focus your eyes is important, keeping your head down is important, estimating how hard to swing is important, being sure the face of the club is facing where the ball should go is important . . . the list goes on. Trying to remember it all is overwhelming!

> Beginners are easy to spot! They walk up to the tee box, put the tee in the ground, and place the ball on top of the tee. Then they "address" the ball and step-by-step do all of the things they know are

important. The overall effect is often jerky and painstakingly long. And, the outcome is that they missed the ball, hit it astray, or sent it a few feet down the fairway. In other words, they appeared awkward and their goal wasn't met. However, by watching tapes, practicing swings, and moving fluidly from one step to the next, this awkwardness can be overcome.

The same can be said for integrating the suggestions in this book into a **fluidity of practice**.

This chapter is designed to provide an example, using a common content area, of how an educator might approach helping learners learn. Think of this as the authors coaching the readers through the various steps so that the anxiety of trying something new is lessened, because the educator has already practiced, in part by valuing the integration of the information conveyed thus far. The intent of this chapter is to help educators visualize how to integrate the previously presented strategies for one learning session.

In this chapter, you will learn, by an example:

1. How to use understanding of self to one's advantage
2. What the importance of serving as role model means for learners
3. How to prepare for the classroom
4. How to create and use agreements
5. How to set the environment
6. How to engage learners
7. How to coach learners
8. How to use questions to promote learning
9. How to construct effective stories
10. When to use standard communication effectively
11. When and how to seek input
12. How to provide feedback

SCENARIO

The following scenario is a compression of what educators do to be effective in the classroom. Not every session needs to be at the intensity of the example here. However, over time, a course can be totally converted to demonstrate effective and engaging strategies.

Context

Rita is a fairly new educator and clearly believes that she is the facilitator, not the fount. Her role, she knows, is to put conditions right so that learning may occur. She has to be knowledgeable, but she knows her job is not to dump what is in her head into those of the learners. Rita has completed some self-assessments, such as the StrengthsFinder, the EQ Map. She also decided to test the Kirton Adaptation-Innovation Inventory (n.d.). She knows that she has a propensity for innovation. Because of this, she is willing to try something different from what her colleagues use in spite of the fact she was presented the "established" course outline. She knows her strengths include learning (from the StrengthsFinder), and that her preferred learning style is applying knowledge in the real world of practice with all of its complexities because she used the Kolb Learning Style Inventory (2005). Rita believes these personal strengths and perspectives will be useful to her as an educator.

At home, Rita may sit around in jeans and a tee shirt, but for days when she is interacting with learners, Rita is always dressed professionally, including representing the dress code of the organization. Rita often wears a lab coat to help learners remember that first she is a nurse. She uses professional language in the classroom, although she understands the current "in" communication and can participate with the best of the learners.

==*FAST FACTS in a NUTSHELL*

- Knowing one's strengths provides a strong starting point in developing greater talents.
- Role modeling being a nurse reinforces for learners what nurses are expected to be.

Preparation Is Key

Today is a planning day. Rita is creating notes, gathering materials, writing questions, practicing various gestures to use in the classroom, and documenting sources. She begins by looking at the syllabus, which she recently revised to provide more dependency on learners coming prepared to learn in the classroom. The following is a general list of what she did:

1. Keeping the same content focus, Rita eliminated the word *lecture* from several of the days' listings of activities. In the areas where she kept the word *lecture* she added other words to convey that it was one of many activities that would be used to promote learning. In each content area, she developed a "Quality and Safety" heading that contained the best practices and key resources learners would need to be able to master the specific area.

2. She created each major topic into a module. Some were designed for online e-learning and validation. Others were designed to create the focus of a classroom session. Both types of modules included a "prep sheet" that laid out some key words, content, recent research, and a description of best practices related to care of patients with certain conditions. These sheets were labeled, "TO BE TURNED IN UPON ENTRY INTO THE CLASS SESSION ON THIS TOPIC (See schedule)." For the online e-learning, the expectation was that the learner submitted this prep sheet

after some readings and thinking time. For the classroom session, the expectation was that this prep sheet was turned in at the door. Individual's names were required on each form.

3. Rita identified recent literature that supported or, in at least one case, refuted the text. Those items were clearly identified in the syllabus and each module always asked for other resources that the learners used, so that Rita was better informed about the quality of their searching efforts.

4. Each classroom session was identified as having more than one learning strategy and they all involved learner participation. Some of the strategies included: interactive notes (which were prepared in advance and were required to be brought to class), video clips illustrating a key point, Internet searches related to the topic of discussion, small group work, and role play. Additionally, Rita had a "plan B" for most activities so that if learners needed more content on a topic, she was immediately prepared with another example and strategy.

To begin her work, Rita creates some notes. These notes include some Post Its™ placed in the syllabus so that she can remember where to access materials. Other notes include reminders to herself, such as a card with the symbols "." and "?" (see Chapter 11, Seeking Input); a card with the notation: "Think/Pair/Square/Share" (Bain, 2004); and a card that says "Check Time."

She gathers materials related to individual sessions and puts them in bags with the date of use noted on the bag. She also gathers materials common to every class session in another bag. For each of the sessions (or as far ahead as she can work before other priorities set in), she writes out at least five questions to ask the group. Currently they are written to specific topics, yet she knows they will eventually become stem questions (ones where specific content can be added but the "stem" remains the same). She can already see one that is a stem question after preparing for two class sessions. She took the two detailed questions and made one stem: "What are the underlying implications of the pathology for _____ (the condition) that this/a patient might experience?"

In addition, Rita has at least two stories to tell during each class sessions. When she told the first one to her colleagues, she could tell they looked bored. Thus, she practiced using her full body to convey her messages. When she said "big," she spread her arms wide to convey the word and opened her eyes widely. Yes, she practiced in front of a mirror so she could see how this looked rather than depending simply on the "feel." She was also aware of the "feel" so that she could depend on it when no mirror was present. She practiced speaking louder and softer to reflect when someone in her story was shouting or whispering. And she leaned forward and cupped her hand around her mouth to convey the whisper. Because her story ended as a surprise, she practiced what that facial expression would look like so that she could remember it for when she told the story in the classroom.

She checked to be sure she had documentation for all of the complex actions required of the nurses so that she could pull those up in the e-library as needed. Rita divided these into two categories, required and recommended, so that she could focus the learners' attention on the most critical information.

Rita pulls a copy of a learning agreement she used in a previous learning session. Rather than simply "plugging" the form into this course, she carefully reviews it to be sure the language fits the level of the learner and that she is comfortable with being able to hold people accountable to what is in the agreement. She knows (self-insight) from a prior experience that she wants to include an agreement about physical space because many learners have different views of what space is theirs. She adds that to the document and decides that because the group may discuss real patients, a statement about confidentiality that reflects various clinical facilities' standards should also be added. Rita also thinks about what types of action she might take if each of the agreements is violated. In fact, she decides to take the agreement and write notes off to the side of at least one strategy she can use for each element if adherence isn't met. Although she often is not a "rules follower," she knows she has to convey the accountability for consequences when something agreed to isn't exhibited in behavior. So, for example, she anticipates the greatest violation to focus on is use of cell phones in class. She identified several actions in increasing order of public acknowledgment:

1. "Let's remember that all cell phones are to be turned off during class."
2. "I hear some conversation on a cell phone. Please turn off the cell phone now."
3. [Approaching an offending learner] "Please step out to the hall and return when you are finished with all of your conversations."
4. "Please leave the classroom and do not reenter until you can continue to commit to your agreement."
5. "We need to discuss the lack of agreement regarding one of our standards…"

Knowing that openings and closings are critical, Rita creates a written statement for the opening to be sure it leads to engaging the learners. For this particular session—one on disruptive behavior in the workplace—Rita poses questions:

- How can we handle abusive coworkers?
- What does abuse look like?
- What resources should we expect in the clinical area to help us deal with abusive peers?

Rita also creates closure statements. This one says: "Most of you will work in zero tolerance workplaces because that is today's expectation. And, many of you will experience a violation of that expectation. Your challenge is to find a method for stopping peer abuse that is comfortable for you. That may be a road less traveled. Thank you for having the courage to change a critical issue for the profession." The closure is designed to inspire action on the part of learners as they engage in the workplace.

Because Rita travels some distance to meet with the group of learners she works with, she checks the online resources about the facility where the learning session will be held. She determines such things as if the furniture is moveable and how many people can be seated comfortably. She knows she doesn't control the number of learners in this onsite learning situation. However, she also knows she can request changes if such are needed for the layout of the furniture. She has a list of learners who are expected in the classroom and she has generated a random list of numbers to create a seating chart and then one for group work. She prints off enough copies for each person so each is clear about who is in the respective small groups. Rita is ready!

FAST FACTS in a NUTSHELL

- Educators who overprepare aren't at a loss of what to do next if the original plan doesn't work.
- Thinking through, and sometimes actually working through, some of the details (e.g., practicing telling a story) prepares the educator to enact elements of facilitating learning.
- Thinking through consequences in advance of using agreements helps educators feel more confident in using them.
- Gathering props, if needed, ahead of time assures that the items will be available when needed.
- Creating agreements helps control the classroom.
- Converting common responses or statements into standard communication allows educators to spend time on other elements of preparation rather than rethinking those responses for each situation.

Implementation

Imagine that Rita has begun her course. She has indicated how the class will operate, she has reviewed and sought concurrence for the agreements, and she has set the expectation of coming prepared to discuss rather than be told something. She was assigned a room that doesn't allow the movement of furniture and she has prepared the group for how small groups, nevertheless, can be formed and used effectively. The following dialogue and details indicate how Rita is actualizing her plan for a greater focus on learning and the learners.

Prior to the beginning of today's session, Rita took her basic materials to the front of the room and made certain the Internet was working in case it was needed. She now stands at what she has designated to the group as the main door and receives the preparation assignment from each learner. She thanks each for submitting the information and if the name is missing on the form, reminds the learner that information is important. As the clock approaches the start time for the class, she closes the door and asks that one of the learners seated near the door collect the remaining papers.

> *Thank you all for submitting your preparation assignment forms. I want to remind you that I posted the big points and questions (with responses from our prior class) to our website. You are making good progress in understanding the complexities of gerontological nursing.* [This is an example of acknowledgment.]

> *We are using the first case study today to form the basis for discussion. What I like about the opportunity we have today is to discuss "gero" from the perspective of the family. We have the daughter who describes herself in ways that match what we call the "sandwich" generation; we have the grandchildren who are committed to so many activities that it is difficult for them to make time for visits with the grandparents. Does this seem "real" for anyone in the room?* (Several hands go up and a short dialogue ensues.) *From what you read in the case study and the literature that relates, what do you believe is the primary nursing concern, and*

> *of course, it has to be supported by a rationale. Thomas, I saw*
> *your hand first. What are you thinking?*

Thomas offers an idea and rationale and then several other learners chime in with mostly similar views. Rita then asks for what else might be seen as an idea and the rationale related to the idea. After one brave soul states an opposing view; Rita coaches that person to say more because the point is valuable and Rita doesn't want the viewpoint dismissed as not valuable. She asks others to provide rationale about how this different view might be valid. Her questions often say only the word "and" with an indication that there is more to think through. Rita then notices that a group in the back of the room is holding a discussion. Rather than pointing this out to the group, Rita simply stops talking and remains still until the group realizes that something different is happening. When they stop talking, Rita moves on.

> *I can see we 'are not all in agreement about this case study.*
> *I have found that to be true in the clinical settings in which I have*
> *worked when insufficient evidence existed to support a definitive*
> *approach. For example, . . .*

Rita launches into a story where she describes clinical experts disagreeing about what is happening for a family. Rather than saying a name and using a passive word such as "said," she changes her voice to portray an older man, a middle-aged woman, and a young child. Rather than using words such as "scold," she shakes her finger as she portrays what the older man is saying to the young child. In short, she is a one-woman show!

She stops abruptly and looks out to the group and says: *"What is going on here?"* And then she says: *"think, pair, square, and share."* The learners instantly know who their partners are and who comprises the square. The syllabus also detailed what to do if a member of the team was absent, so that the usual "I don't have a partner" responses were avoided. As the process concludes, Rita then provides the group with some feedback about what is actually going on in the case study and how the nurses in the story came to conclusions that were helpful. As Rita moves on, she notices the same group of learners who had an earlier sidebar conversation are engaged in another private discussion. Rather than simply stopping, this time Rita says, "*I note that we are not all living within the class agreements with which we concurred. If a conversation unrelated to the topic needs to be held, please step into the hall and come back when you are done.*" From an earlier discussion about agreements, the learners know that the next time this happens, Rita will stop the discussion and ask the specific members of the group to step outside. Initially learners were concerned about the consequences, as was Rita. Publicly calling out behavior seemed unfair to the learners; however, they quickly agreed that if they put this behavior in the context of how to hold others accountable, it would also be a useful lesson for them to use clinically. All of this activity thus far has been designed to engage the learner in being an active participant in the learning situation.

Meanwhile someone's cell phone rings. Through prior agreement, Rita has indicated she will say "*cell phone*" and that message would connote that one of the agreements about cell phone usage was being violated. This agreed upon, standard communication allows Rita to short cut a longer conversation about cell phone usage. If the behavior continues with that learner or other learners have ringing phones, Rita knows she will need to stop the discussion and focus on the agreements and what they mean.

With a few minutes left to class, Rita thanks the learners for their participation and points out that they all are doing well with the responses related to the physical aspects of aging. What learners need more work on is the psychosocial aspect. Thus, Rita goes to "plan B" and indicates that another case study with different references will be available by the end of the day so that learners can develop greater insights into the psychosocial aspects. Then Rita calls for the Big Point/Big Question and learners take out a piece of paper and write the words *POINT* and *QUESTION* and record their thoughts. Rita moves to the back of the room and collects the papers as the learners leave. She thanks the learners for being present in the discussion. Rita goes to her laptop, pulls up the "Plan B" file for the class session, and transmits the psychosocial case study to the web site.

═══════════════════════════════════*FAST FACTS in a NUTSHELL*

- Spending time at the beginning of any interaction to set the stage for how the interaction will evolve allows "shorthand" communication during the session.
- Expecting that learners will arrive with evidence of work done in preparation not only facilitates the classroom discussion, but also fosters valuable professional behaviors.
- Having questions and stories for the major content areas allows the educator to focus on learning for the real world.
- The effective use of standard communication conveys a sense of fairness to learners.
- Sometimes coaching can be as simple as saying the word "and."

Reflection

Rita gathers her materials and goes to a small, quiet space. She quickly jots a few notes about how class went today and what she can do to improve the learning situation for next time. Because she started this class session with a case study and she now knows learners need more support with the psychosocial aspects of care, she writes the opening statement for the next class session, using an anticipation strategy (see Chapter 6, Engaging the Learners). She writes: "*Today we are going to look at a guaranteed method for dealing with anxious patients. It is a strategy you'll love. It's the best thing I've found and the literature supports its use.*"

She reflects on how she handled the classroom disruptions. She acknowledges to herself that she hates to "reprimand" people and that she needs to reframe her thinking to see this as role modeling by holding others accountable. She now has the insight that if this is hard for her—a seasoned professional—new nurses will have this struggle too. She writes how she feels about this inner conflict so that at some point she can share this with others to acknowledge that accountability is challenging.

Because several questions were asked about some basic information related to the case study, Rita makes notes about what to add to it and also makes a note to check future case studies. Further, as a member of AACN (American Association of Critical Care Nurses), Rita accesses the members-only information to determine if there are resources that would be useful to her in working with geriatric patients. She also checks the site for the National Gerontological Nursing Association and makes a note to consider joining this association too.

Rita realizes that she didn't capitalize on the learners who were least likely to be engaged (back of the room). She places a note on a piece of paper that says: "CHECK THE BACK OF THE ROOM." Then she realizes that if she looks there and the learners are not engaged, she will need to do something. She creates an example of getting to stable datum (see Chapter 6, Engaging the Learners) for three critical points in the next session.

Rita also reflects on how she felt when she was portraying different people. She ponders that for a bit and decides to download some movies where one of the stars portrays other characters to learn from how that portrayal looks. She knows there just aren't enough hours in the day to practice any presentation several times.

Rita believes she is making progress as an educator. Yet, she decides to explore learning opportunities to help her achieve excellence in the classroom. Her goal is to be her best!

Finally, she reflects on whether or not she is using her knowledge of herself. She asks herself if she is doing what she does best and if not, how she can modify what she must do to capitalize on her strengths and perspectives. Thinking ahead, she considers whether she is willing to have learners review a test in class or if she wants to build some review based on the item analysis information she will receive. She is aware that if she decides not to conduct a review, there may be some pushback. She thinks about what standard messages might be needed to explain consistently her rationale for her action.

She then thinks in the "bigger picture" perspective and considers if she has role modeled being a nurse to the extent that learners could envision themselves as nurses too. During this process, she asks herself what might happen if she told the group about role modeling and asked for feedback.

Finally, she makes a checklist of strategies she knows or has learned and decides to be sure to use at least two in every learning encounter to capitalize on how learners best learn. She also knows that varying how she uses these strategies will strengthen her understanding of them and provide her with other elements to include in her repertoire.

After all of this, Rita decides that the class session went fairly well and that it was fairly effective. She turns to the Big Point and Big Question papers and summarizes them to post to the online portion of the course so that learners have this feedback prior to the next class session. Rita glances at her phone and sees that she needs to wrap up this session in order to meet her next obligation. She writes the word *Effective* beside the class date to remind herself that things did go well and that learning was fairly effective. She already knows the improvements she needs to address.

═══════════════════*FAST FACTS in a NUTSHELL*

- Taking time to reflect on any learner interaction allows educators to provide self-feedback to improve their teaching.
- Documenting needed changes at that time allows for greater clarity about what to do rather than waiting until the next time the session is to be offered.

SYNTHESIS

By planning ahead, Rita was able to think through during a calm time what she might do or say when the stress of a classroom situation might prevent her from thinking so clearly. Making reminders of things to check and thinking about specific responses to violations of agreements gave Rita a sense of confidence rather than a sense of surprise when something didn't work quite right. Practicing, even if only for the more complex things such as storytelling, allowed Rita to feel more at ease and "know" what she looked like when she made certain facial expressions or body gestures. She knew she wouldn't always be able to have this rehearsal time and she knew to pay attention to the feel of something so she could transfer that experience to another situation. Thinking through how holding people accountable is a higher professional value than avoiding conflict allowed Rita to call to the attention of certain learners their violation of some of the agreements.

By reflecting after the teaching activity, Rita was able to consider if she needed to do something different and if so, what that might be. It allowed her to value the work she had done and define specific strategies to improve. Rita knew she had not used all of the strategies available to her and she acknowledged that the intensity of using too many would be too overwhelming for the average class session. However, she also knew she had other resources readily available (or was seeking them) so that she would continue to develop as a highly competent, engaged educator.

Finally, Rita—and all of us—can acknowledge that pre-planning and reflecting are critical to our success as educators. Creating classroom interactions that transport learners to clinical experiences promotes the essence of nursing, capitalizes on the expertise of educators, and focuses on becoming expert at learning. These are the goals of nurse educators.

References

Bain, K. (2004). *What the best college teachers do.* Cambridge, MA: Harvard University Press.

Benner, P., Sutphen, M., Leonard, V., & Day, L. (2010). *Educating nurses: A call for radical transformation.* San Francisco, CA: Jossey-Bass.

Berwick, D. (2006). *5 million lives campaign.* Retrieved from http://www.ihi.org/offerings/Initiatives/PastStrategicInitiatives/5Million LivesCampaign/Pages/default.aspx

Bradberry, T., & Greaves, J. (2009). *Emotional Intelligence 2.0.* San Diego, CA: TalentSmart.

Caputi, L. (2010). *Teaching Nursing: The Art and Science.* Vol. 3 (2nd ed.). Dupage, WI: College of DuPage.

Cronenwelt, L., Sherwood, G., Barnsteiner, J., Disch, J., Johnson, J., Mitchell, P., . . . Warren, J. (2007). Quality and safety education for nurses. *Nursing Outlook, 55*(3), 122–131.

Donner, G. J., & Wheeler, M. M. (2009). *Coaching in nursing: An introduction.* Indianapolis, IN: International Council of Nurses and the Honor Society of Nursing, Sigma Theta Tau International.

Dukette, D., & Cornish, D. (2009). *The essential 20: Twenty components of an excellent health care team* (pp. 72–73). Pittsburgh, PA: RoseDog Books.

Essi Systems. (n.d.). *EQ Map Online.* Retrieved from www.eqmapon line.com

Goleman, D., Boyatzis, R., & McKee, A. (2002). *Primal leadership: Realizing the power of emotional intelligence.* Boston, MA: Harvard Business School.

Guber, P. (2011). *Tell to win: Connect, persuade, and triumph with the hidden power of story.* New York, NY: Crown Business.

Guinness, O. (1999). *Character counts: Leadership qualities in Washington, Wilberforce, Lincoln, and Solzhenitsyn.* Grand Rapids, MI: Baker Books.

Hurlock, E. (1977). *Child Development.* (6th ed.) MaGrawHill, TX: MaGraw-Hill.

International Coach Federation. (n.d.). *ICF code of ethics.* Retrieved from www.coachfederation.org/about-icf/ethics/icf-code-of-ethics

Kirton Adaptation-Innovation Inventory. (n.d.). Retrieved from www.kaicentre.com

Koegel, T. J. (2007). *The exceptional presenter: A proven formula to open up! and own the room.* Austin, TX: Greenleaf.

Kohn, L., Corrigan, J. M., & Donaldson, M. S. (2000). *To err is human: Building a safer health system.* Washington, DC: National Academies Press.

Kolb, A. Y., & Kolb, D. A. (2005). *The Kolb Learning Style Inventory, Version 3.1.* Retrieved from www.whitewater-rescue.com/support/pagepics/lsitechmanual.pdf

Kowalski, K. (2009a). More situations in which questions are valuable. *The Journal of Continuing Education in Nursing: Continuing Competence for the Future, 40*(9), 393.

Kowalski, K. (2009b). Situations in which questions are valuable. *The Journal of Continuing Education in Nursing: Continuing Competence for the Future, 40*(8), 344–345.

Liesveld, R., & Miller, J. A. (2005). *Teach with your strengths: How great teachers inspire their students.* New York, NY: Gallup Press.

Light, R. J. (1986). *Strengthening colleges and universities: The Harvard Assessment Seminars.* Retrieved from http://net.educause.edu/ir/library/pdf/ff0603S.pdf

Pisanos, D. (2011). Emotional intelligence: It's more than IQ. *The Journal of Continuing Education in Nursing: Continuing Competence for the Future, 42*(10), 439–440.

Rath, T. (2007). *StrengthsFinder 2.0.* New York, NY: Gallup Press.

Rose, C., & Nicholl, M. J. (1997). *Accelerated learning for the 21st century.* New York, NY: Dell.

Scriven, M. (1967). The methodology of evaluation. In R. W. Tyler, R. M. Gagne, & M. Scriven (Eds.), *Perspectives of curriculum evaluation* (pp. 39–83). Chicago, IL: Rand McNally.

Yoder-Wise, P. S. (2010). More serendipity: The Winkler County Trial. *The Journal of Continuing Education in Nursing: Continuing Competence for the Future, 41*(3), 147.

Yoder-Wise, P. S., & Kowalski, K. (2006). *Beyond leading and managing: Nursing administration for the future* (p. 131). St. Louis, MO: Elsevier.

Index

Printed in the United States
By Bookmasters